Advances in Preterm Delivery

Advances in Preterm Delivery

Editor

Eyal Sheiner

MDPI • Basel • Beijing • Wuhan • Barcelona • Belgrade • Manchester • Tokyo • Cluj • Tianjin

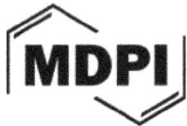

Editor
Eyal Sheiner
Soroka University Medical
Center
Israel

Editorial Office
MDPI
St. Alban-Anlage 66
4052 Basel, Switzerland

This is a reprint of articles from the Special Issue published online in the open access journal *Journal of Clinical Medicine* (ISSN 2077-0383) (available at: https://www.mdpi.com/journal/jcm/special_issues/Advances_Preterm_Delivery).

For citation purposes, cite each article independently as indicated on the article page online and as indicated below:

LastName, A.A.; LastName, B.B.; LastName, C.C. Article Title. *Journal Name* **Year**, *Volume Number*, Page Range.

ISBN 978-3-0365-4751-0 (Hbk)
ISBN 978-3-0365-4752-7 (PDF)

© 2022 by the authors. Articles in this book are Open Access and distributed under the Creative Commons Attribution (CC BY) license, which allows users to download, copy and build upon published articles, as long as the author and publisher are properly credited, which ensures maximum dissemination and a wider impact of our publications.

The book as a whole is distributed by MDPI under the terms and conditions of the Creative Commons license CC BY-NC-ND.

Contents

About the Editor vii

Tamar Wainstock and Eyal Sheiner
"Advances in Preterm Delivery"—How Can We Advance Further?
Reprinted from: *J. Clin. Med.* **2022**, *11*, 3436, doi:10.3390/jcm11123436 1

Erez Tsumi, Itai Hazan, Tamir Regev, Samuel Leeman, Chiya Barrett, Noa Fried Regev and Eyal Sheiner
The Association between Gestational Age and Risk for Long Term Ophthalmic Morbidities among Offspring Delivered in Different Preterm Subgroups
Reprinted from: *J. Clin. Med.* **2022**, *11*, 2562, doi:10.3390/jcm11092562 5

Tamar Wainstock and Eyal Sheiner
Low Five-Minute Apgar Score and Neurological Morbidities: Does Prematurity Modify the Association?
Reprinted from: *J. Clin. Med.* **2022**, *11*, 1922, doi:10.3390/jcm11071922 19

Gil Gutvirtz, Tamar Wainstock, Eyal Sheiner and Gali Pariente
Prematurity and Long-Term Respiratory Morbidity—What Is the Critical Gestational Age Threshold?
Reprinted from: *J. Clin. Med.* **2022**, *11*, 751, doi:10.3390/jcm11030751 29

Natalia Saldaña-García, María Gracia Espinosa-Fernández, Celia Gómez-Robles, Antonio Javier Postigo-Jiménez, Nicholas Bello, Francisca Rius-Díaz and Tomás Sánchez-Tamayo
Benefits of a Single Dose of Betamethasone in Imminent Preterm Labour
Reprinted from: *J. Clin. Med.* **2022**, *11*, 20, doi:10.3390/jcm11010020 43

Izabela Dymanowska-Dyjak, Aleksandra Stupak, Adrianna Kondracka, Tomasz Geca, Arkadiusz Krzyżanowski and Anna Kwaśniewska
Elastography and Metalloproteinases in Patients at High Risk of Preterm Labor
Reprinted from: *J. Clin. Med.* **2021**, *10*, 3886, doi:10.3390/jcm10173886 53

Dora Davidov, Eyal Sheiner, Tamar Wainstock, Shayna Miodownik and Gali Pariente
Maternal Systemic Lupus Erythematosus (SLE) High Risk for Preterm Delivery and Not for Long-Term Neurological Morbidity of the Offspring
Reprinted from: *J. Clin. Med.* **2021**, *10*, 2952, doi:10.3390/jcm10132952 75

Shiran Zer, Tamar Wainstock, Eyal Sheiner, Shayna Miodownik and Gali Pariente
Identifying the Critical Threshold for Long-Term Pediatric Neurological Hospitalizations of the Offspring in Preterm Delivery
Reprinted from: *J. Clin. Med.* **2021**, *10*, 2919, doi:10.3390/ jcm10132919 83

Dvora Kluwgant, Tamar Wainstock, Eyal Sheiner and Gali Pariente
Preterm Delivery; Who Is at Risk?
Reprinted from: *J. Clin. Med.* **2021**, *10*, 2279, doi:10.3390/jcm10112279 95

Tamar Wainstock, Ruslan Sergienko and Eyal Sheiner
Can We Predict Preterm Delivery Based on the Previous Pregnancy?
Reprinted from: *J. Clin. Med.* **2021**, *10*, 1517, doi:10.3390/jcm10071517 107

Monica Di Paola, Viola Seravalli, Sara Paccosi, Carlotta Linari, Astrid Parenti, Carlotta De Filippo, Michele Tanturli, Francesco Vitali, Maria Gabriella Torcia and Mariarosaria Di Tommaso
Identification of Vaginal Microbial Communities Associated with Extreme Cervical Shortening in Pregnant Women
Reprinted from: *J. Clin. Med.* **2020**, *9*, 3621, doi:10.3390/jcm9113621 . . . . **117**

Gian Carlo Di Renzo, Valentina Tosto, Valentina Tsibizova and Eduardo Fonseca
Prevention of Preterm Birth with Progesterone
Reprinted from: *J. Clin. Med.* **2021**, *10*, 4511, doi:10.3390/jcm10194511 . . . . **133**

About the Editor

Eyal Sheiner

Eyal Sheiner, MD, PhD, is a Deichmann-Lerner Full Professor. He is the Chairman of the Department of Obstetrics and Gynecology B at the Soroka University Medical Center, Beer-Sheva, Israel, and the Vice Dean, Academic Promotion, Faculty of Health Sciences, Ben-Gurion University of the Negev.

Prof. Sheiner is in charge of the final examinations for Ob/Gyn residents in Israel, the head of the Southern Ob/Gyn branch, and a selected member of the Israeli National Academy of Science in Medicine, under the Israeli Medical Associations. Previously, he served as the Director of the Residency Program and as the Deputy Director General of the Soroka University Medical Center.

His PhD study and ultrasound fellowship at the Rush University Medical Center (Chicago, Il) were supported by a grant from the Fulbright Visiting Scholar Program of the United States. Professor Sheiner has published extensively in the area of perinatal epidemiology, and has more than 600 peer-reviewed publications. He led the FIGO postpregnancy initiative guidelines. He is the editor of ten books and a member of the Editorial Boards of six scientific journals.

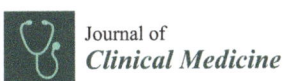

Editorial

"Advances in Preterm Delivery"—How Can We Advance Further?

Tamar Wainstock [1] and Eyal Sheiner [2,*]

[1] Department of Public Health, Faculty of Health Sciences, Ben-Gurion University of the Negev, Beer-Sheva 8410501, Israel; wainstoc@bgu.ac.il
[2] Department of Obstetrics and Gynecology, Soroka University Medical Center, Ben-Gurion University of the Negev, Beer-Sheva 8410501, Israel
* Correspondence: sheiner@bgu.ac.il

Preterm delivery (PTD: <37 gestational weeks) complicates 5–13% of deliveries worldwide [1], and is a leading cause of perinatal and childhood mortality and morbidity [2–5]. PTD is also a risk factor for long-term maternal health complications, including cardiovascular and renal morbidities [6,7].

In most countries, PTD rates are increasing, and an annual estimation of 15 million babies, which equates to 11.1% of live births, are born prematurely worldwide [8].

Spontaneous preterm parturition is a result of the pathological activation of one or more of the processes leading to delivery. The etiology of spontaneous preterm labor, which accounts for 70–83% of PTDs, is mostly unknown [9,10], and multiple etiologies are usually involved; these include cervical insufficiency, uterine ischemia, intrauterine infections, prior cervical surgeries, a decline in progesterone action (a critical hormone in pregnancy maintenance), uterine malformations, and others. Iatrogenic PTD may be indicated in cases of possible hazard to the mother or the fetus, mainly due to preeclampsia, fetal distress, or severe intrauterine growth restriction [11]. In addition to the differentiation between spontaneous or indicated, PTD can be categorized based on gestational age at delivery as follows: extreme preterm (<28 gestational weeks), very preterm (28–<32 gestational weeks), moderate preterm (32–<34 gestational weeks), and late preterm (34–<37 complete gestational weeks), the latter of which is when most PTDs occur [12].

Prevention strategies have been suggested and practiced to lower the risk of PTD; however, their effectiveness is questioned, especially among women considered to be at low risk for PTD [13–15]. These strategies may include progesterone administration, cervical cerclage, or antibiotic treatment.

Risk factors for PTD are obstetrical, socio-economical, behavioral, environmental, and genetic, and include young or old maternal age, infertility treatments, and smoking [16,17]. For instance, in this Special Issue, Kluwgant et al. mentions the high risk of extreme PTD among women with a history of placental abruption, placenta previa, and multiple gestation. Studies have shown variations in the effect size of the different risk factors based on the PTD type (spontaneous or indicated) and whether the case is initial PTD or recurrent PTD [18,19]. Studies addressing risk factors for PTD by type of PTD are presented in this Special Issue [16,18]. The leading risk factor for PTD is having a history of PTDs [19,20]; moreover, the risk increases with each additional PTD, or if the PTD occurred in the immediately preceding pregnancy, and if the gestational age of the first PTD was earlier [21]. The risk of recurrent spontaneous PTD varies among studies, from 18–31.6% [22,23].

One of the early detectable PTD risk factors is cervical shortening or insufficiency (cervical length ≤ 25 mm), defined as an inability of the cervix to remain closed during pregnancy [24]. However, cervical length was found to have a low predictive value, as only a small fraction of women with spontaneous preterm birth had a short cervix, and only

Citation: Wainstock, T.; Sheiner, E. "Advances in Preterm Delivery"—How Can We Advance Further? *J. Clin. Med.* **2022**, *11*, 3436. https://doi.org/10.3390/jcm11123436

Received: 7 June 2022
Accepted: 13 June 2022
Published: 15 June 2022

Publisher's Note: MDPI stays neutral with regard to jurisdictional claims in published maps and institutional affiliations.

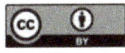

Copyright: © 2022 by the authors. Licensee MDPI, Basel, Switzerland. This article is an open access article distributed under the terms and conditions of the Creative Commons Attribution (CC BY) license (https://creativecommons.org/licenses/by/4.0/).

half of those with a short cervix delivered prematurely [25]. Recurrent PTD, however, is more strongly associated with cervical length in the subsequent pregnancy, and it has a higher predictive value in recurrent compared to initial PTD [24,25].

Since PTD events are likely to re-occur in the same mother and within the family [26], factors that are persistent, such as genetic factors, or factors which are present over a long time span, such as exposure to environmental factors, are likely involved in PTD re-occurrence. Indeed, exposure to environmental factors such as smoking and air pollution have been associated with an increased risk of recurrent PTD [27,28]. Genetic studies based on whole-exome sequencing suggested an association between PTD and inflammatory regulation genes [29], as well as genes related to estrogen receptor alteration [30]. Although genetic factors have been associated with PTD risk, this has not been studied in association with recurrent PTD risk.

Fetal development occurs throughout the entire pregnancy until full term; therefore, when PTD occurs, the newborn is not physiologically and metabolically mature, leading to immediate and long-term complications [2–5]. The severity of these complications depends mainly on gestational age at delivery, and increases with reduced gestational age; this is reported by Gutvirtz et al. [3] and Zer at al. [4] in our Special Issue, in their works regarding risk of prematurity and respiratory or neurologic morbidities in offspring. In a large retrospective cohort, Gutvirtz et al. [3] found that offspring born at an extremely premature gestational age were ~3 times more likely to be hospitalized with respiratory morbidities, and Zer at al. [4] found that they were ~3.9 times more likely to be hospitalized with neurologic morbidities, compared to offspring born at term. Besides immediate and long-term health effects, PTD entails great economic consequences due to health costs, and the support of families and their offspring throughout life; this begins with the immediate hospitalization and intensive care treatment upon delivery. Aspects of the special treatment of premature newborns are also presented in this Special Issue by Saldana-Garcia et al. [31], who address the benefits of early interventions in reducing respiratory-related risk to the newborn. In the United States, the annual costs associated with PTD in the year 2005 were USD 26.2 billion [32].

Lowering the rate of this major, relatively prevalent pregnancy complication has been declared by the WHO as "an urgent priority for reaching Millennium Development Goal 4, calling for the reduction of child deaths" [33]. Although women with a history of PTD are clearly a population at risk for a subsequent PTD, and although strategies to prevent preterm birth have been practiced for over 30 years, the expectations have not been met, and PTD rates have not declined. Some PTD risk factors are preventable, and addressing them at the personal (e.g., patient education regarding prenatal product consumption and smoking) and population levels (e.g., industries and legislation), may decrease PTD incidence. Environmental policy has the potential to reduce PTD; this has recently been shown in the US, where legislation and health concerns have led to the closure of coal and oil power plants, and to the lowering of PTD incidence [34]. Even a small reduction in PTD incidence may have a large public-health and economic impact, in terms of preventing perinatal mortality, morbidity, and lifelong disability among affected infants.

We would like to give special thanks to the colleagues who took part in this project for their valuable contributions.

Author Contributions: Conceptualization, T.W. and E.S.; methodology, T.W. and E.S.; data curation, T.W. and E.S.; writing—original draft preparation, T.W.; review and editing, E.S. All authors have read and agreed to the published version of the manuscript.

Funding: This research received no external funding.

Conflicts of Interest: The authors declare no conflict of interest.

References

1. WHO. Available online: http://www.who.int/topics/preterm_birth/en/ (accessed on 14 June 2022).
2. Ohana, O.; Wainstock, T.; Sheiner, E.; Leibson, T.; Pariente, G. Long-term digestive hospitalizations of premature infants (besides necrotizing enterocolitis): Is there a critical threshold? *Arch. Gynecol. Obstet.* **2021**, *304*, 455–463. [CrossRef]
3. Gutvirtz, G.; Wainstock, T.; Sheiner, E.; Pariente, G. Prematurity and Long-Term Respiratory Morbidity-What Is the Critical Gestational Age Threshold? *J. Clin. Med.* **2022**, *11*, 751. [CrossRef]
4. Zer, S.; Wainstock, T.; Sheiner, E.; Miodownik, S.; Pariente, G. Identifying the Critical Threshold for Long-Term Pediatric Neurological Hospitalizations of the Offspring in Preterm Delivery. *J. Clin. Med.* **2021**, *10*, 2919. [CrossRef]
5. Tsumi, E.; Hazan, I.; Regev, T.; Leeman, S.; Barrett, C.; Fried Regev, N.; Sheiner, E. The Association between Gestational Age and Risk for Long Term Ophthalmic Morbidities among Offspring Delivered in Different Preterm Subgroups. *J. Clin. Med.* **2022**, *11*, 2562. [CrossRef]
6. Pariente, G.; Kessous, R.; Sergienko, R.; Sheiner, E. Is preterm delivery an independent risk factor for long-term maternal kidney disease? *J. Matern. Fetal Neonatal Med.* **2017**, *30*, 1102–1107. [CrossRef]
7. Kessous, R.; Shoham-Vardi, I.; Pariente, G.; Holcberg, G.; Sheiner, E. An association between preterm delivery and long-term maternal cardiovascular morbidity. *Am. J. Obstet. Gynecol.* **2013**, *209*, 368.e1–368.e8. [CrossRef]
8. Blencowe, H.; Cousens, S.; Chou, D.; Oestergaard, M.; Say, L.; Moller, A.B.; Kinney, M.; Lawn, J. Born Too Soon Preterm Birth Action Group: The global epidemiology of 15 million preterm births. *Reprod. Health* **2013**, *10* (Suppl. 1), S2. [CrossRef]
9. Goldenberg, R.L.; Culhane, J.F.; Iams, J.D.; Romero, R. Epidemiology and causes of preterm birth. *Lancet* **2008**, *371*, 75–84. [CrossRef]
10. Ananth, C.V.; Getahun, D.; Peltier, M.R.; Salihu, H.M.; Vintzileos, A.M. Recurrence of spontaneous versus medically indicated preterm birth. *Am. J. Obstet. Gynecol.* **2006**, *195*, 643–650. [CrossRef]
11. Ananth, C.V.; Vintzileos, A.M. Maternal-fetal conditions necessitating a medical intervention resulting in preterm birth. *Am. J. Obstet. Gynecol.* **2006**, *195*, 1557–1563. [CrossRef]
12. Kramer, M.S.; Papageorghiou, A.; Culhane, J.; Bhutta, Z.; Goldenberg, R.L.; Gravett, M.; Iams, J.D.; Conde-Agudelo, A.; Waller, S.; Barros, F.; et al. Challenges in defining and classifying the preterm birth syndrome. *Am. J. Obstet. Gynecol.* **2012**, *206*, 108–112. [CrossRef]
13. Berghella, V.; Rafael, T.J.; Szychowski, J.M.; Rust, O.A.; Owen, J. Cerclage for short cervix on ultrasonography in women with singleton gestations and previous preterm birth: A meta-analysis. *Obstet. Gynecol.* **2011**, *117*, 6636–6671. [CrossRef]
14. Romero, R.; Yeo, L.; Chaemsaithong, P.; Chaiworapongsa, T.; Hassan, S.S. Progesterone to prevent spontaneous preterm birth. *Semin. Fetal Neonatal Med.* **2014**, *19*, 15–26. [CrossRef]
15. da Fonseca, E.B.; Bittar, R.E.; Carvalho, M.H.; Zugaib, M. Prophylactic administration of progesterone by vaginal suppository to reduce the incidence of spontaneous preterm birth in women at increased risk: A randomized placebo-controlled double-blind study. *Am. J. Obstet. Gynecol.* **2003**, *188*, 419–424. [CrossRef]
16. Kluwgant, D.; Wainstock, T.; Sheiner, E.; Pariente, G. Preterm Delivery; Who Is at Risk? *J. Clin. Med.* **2021**, *10*, 2279. [CrossRef]
17. Grantz, K.L.; Hinkle, S.N.; Mendola, P.; Sjaarda, L.A.; Leishear, K.; Albert, P.S. Differences in risk factors for recurrent versus incident preterm delivery. *Am. J. Epidemio.* **2015**, *182*, 157–167. [CrossRef]
18. Asrat, T.; Lewis, D.F.; Garite, T.J.; Major, C.A.; Nageotte, M.P.; Towers, C.V.; Montgomery, D.M.; Dorchester, W.A. Rate of recurrence of preterm premature rupture of membranes in consecutive pregnancies. *Am. J. Obstet. Gynecol.* **1991**, *165*, 1111–1115. [CrossRef]
19. Yang, J.; Baer, R.J.; Berghella, V.; Chambers, C.; Chung, P.; Coker, T.; Currier, R.J.; Druzin, M.L.; Kuppermann, M.; Muglia, L.J.; et al. Recurrence of Preterm Birth and Early Term Birth. *Obstet. Gynecol.* **2016**, *128*, 364–372. [CrossRef]
20. Mercer, B.M.; Goldenberg, R.L.; Moawad, A.H.; Meis, P.J.; Iams, J.D.; Das, A.F.; Caritis, S.N.; Miodovnik, M.; Menard, M.K.; Thurnau, G.R.; et al. The preterm prediction study: Effect of gestational age and cause of preterm birth on subsequent obstetric outcome. National Institute of Child Health and Human Development Maternal-Fetal Medicine Units Network. *Am. J. Obstet. Gynecol.* **1999**, *181*, 1216–1221. [CrossRef]
21. Carr-Hill, R.A.; Hall, M.H. The repetition of spontaneous preterm labour. *Br. J. Obstet. Gynaecol.* **1985**, *92*, 921–928. [CrossRef]
22. Laughon, S.K.; Albert, P.S.; Leishear, K.; Mendola, P. The NICHD Consecutive Pregnancies Study: Recurrent preterm delivery by subtype. *Am. J. Obstet. Gynecol.* **2014**, *210*, 131.e1–131.e1318. [CrossRef] [PubMed]
23. Grant, A. Cervical cerclage to prolong pregnancy. In *Effective Care in Pregnancy and Childbirth*; Chalmers, I., Enkin, M., Keirse, M.J.N.C., Eds.; Oxford University Press: New York, NY, USA, 1989; Volume 1, pp. 633–646.
24. Mazaki-Tovi, S.; Romero, R.; Kusanovic, J.P.; Erez, O.; Pineles, B.L.; Gotsch, F.; Mittal, P.; Than, N.G.; Espinoza, J.; Hassan, S.S. Recurrent preterm birth. *Semin. Perinatol.* **2007**, *31*, 142–158. [CrossRef] [PubMed]
25. Iams, J.D.; Goldenberg, R.L.; Mercer, B.M.; Moawad, A.; Thom, E.; Meis, P.J.; McNellis, D.; Caritis, S.N.; Miodovnik, M.; Menard, M.K.; et al. The Preterm Prediction Study: Recurrence risk of spontaneous preterm birth. National Institute of Child Health and Human Development Maternal-Fetal Medicine Units Network. *Am. J. Obstet. Gynecol.* **1998**, *178*, 1035–1040. [CrossRef]
26. Sherf, Y.; Sheiner, E.; Vardi, I.S.; Sergienko, R.; Klein, J.; Bilenko, N. Recurrence of Preterm Delivery in Women with a Family History of Preterm Delivery. *Am. J. Perinatol.* **2017**, *34*, 397–402. [CrossRef] [PubMed]
27. Cnattingius, S.; Granath, F.; Petersson, G.; Harlow, B.L. The influence of gestational age and smoking habits on the risk of subsequent preterm deliveries. *N. Engl. J. Med.* **1999**, *341*, 943–948. [CrossRef]

28. Li, Q.; Wang, Y.Y.; Guo, Y.; Zhou, H.; Wang, X.; Wang, Q.; Shen, H.; Zhang, Y.; Yan, D.; Zhang, Y.; et al. Effect of airborne particulate matter of 2.5 μm or less on preterm birth: A national birth cohort study in China. *Environ. Int.* **2018**, *121 Pt 2*, 1128–1136. [CrossRef]
29. Strauss, J.F., III.; Romero, R.; Gomez-Lopez, N.; Haymond-Thornburg, H.; Modi, B.P.; Teves, M.E.; Pearson, L.N.; York, T.P.; Schenkein, H.A. Spontaneous preterm birth: Advances toward the discovery of genetic predisposition. *Am. J. Obstet. Gynecol.* **2018**, *218*, 294–314.e2. [CrossRef]
30. Zhang, G.; Feenstra, B.; Bacelis, J.; Liu, X.; Muglia, L.M.; Juodakis, J.; Miller, D.E.; Litterman, N.; Jiang, P.P.; Russell, L.; et al. Genetic Associations with Gestational Duration and Spontaneous Preterm Birth. *N. Engl. J. Med.* **2017**, *377*, 1156–1167. [CrossRef]
31. Saldaña-García, N.; Espinosa-Fernández, M.G.; Martínez-Pajares, J.D.; Tapia-Moreno, E.; Moreno-Samos, M.; Cuenca-Marín, C.; Rius-Díaz, F.; Sánchez-Tamayo, T. Antenatal Betamethasone Every 12 Hours in Imminent Preterm Labour. *J. Clin. Med.* **2022**, *11*, 1227. [CrossRef]
32. Behrman, R.E.; Adashi, E.Y.; Allen, M.C. *Committee on Understanding Premature Birth and Assuring Health Outcomes Board on Health Sciences Policy, Preterm Birth: Causes, Consequences and Prevention*; The National Academies Press: Washington, DC, USA, 2006.
33. Available online: https://www.un.org/millenniumgoals/2015_MDG_Report/pdf/MDG%202015%20PR%20Key%20Facts%20Global.pdf (accessed on 14 June 2022).
34. Casey, J.A.; Karasek, D.; Ogburn, E.L.; Goin, D.E.; Dang, K.; Braveman, P.A.; Morello-Frosch, R. Retirements of Coal and Oil Power Plants in California: Association with Reduced Preterm Birth Among Populations Nearby. *Am. J. Epidemiol.* **2018**, *187*, 1586–1594. [CrossRef]

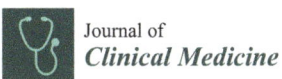

Article

The Association between Gestational Age and Risk for Long Term Ophthalmic Morbidities among Offspring Delivered in Different Preterm Subgroups

Erez Tsumi [1,*,†], Itai Hazan [2,†], Tamir Regev [1], Samuel Leeman [1], Chiya Barrett [1], Noa Fried Regev [3] and Eyal Sheiner [4,*]

1. Department of Ophthalmology, Soroka University Medical Center, Ben-Gurion University of the Negev, Beer-Sheva 8410101, Israel; tamirre@clalit.org.il (T.R.); leemans@post.bgu.ac.il (S.L.); barat@post.bgu.ac.il (C.B.)
2. Joyce and Irving Goldman Medical School, Faculty of Health Sciences, Ben-Gurion University of the Negev, Beer-Sheva 8410501, Israel; itaihaz@post.bgu.ac.il
3. Department of Emergency Medicine, Soroka University Medical Center, Ben-Gurion University of the Negev, Beer-Sheva 8410101, Israel; noafri@clalit.org.il
4. Department of Obstetrics and Gynecology, Soroka University Medical Center, Ben-Gurion University of the Negev, Beer-Sheva 8410101, Israel
* Correspondence: ertsumi@post.bgu.ac.il (E.T.); sheiner@bgu.ac.il (E.S.)
† These authors contributed equally to this paper.

Abstract: Objective: To investigate whether there is a linear association between the degree of prematurity and the risk for long-term ophthalmic morbidity among preterm infants. Study design: A population-based, retrospective cohort study, which included all singleton deliveries occurring between 1991 and 2014 at a single tertiary medical center. All infants were divided into four groups according to gestational age categories: extremely preterm births, very preterm births, moderate to late preterm births and term deliveries (reference group). Hospitalizations of offspring up to 18 years of age involving ophthalmic morbidity were evaluated. Survival curves compared cumulative hospitalizations and regression models controlled for confounding variables. Results: During the study period, 243,363 deliveries met the inclusion criteria. Ophthalmic-related hospitalization rates were lower among children born at term (0.9%) as compared with extremely preterm (3.6%), very preterm (2%), and moderate to late preterm (1.4%) born offspring ($p < 0.01$; using the chi-square test for trends). The survival curve demonstrated significantly different hospitalization rates between the gestational ages ($p < 0.001$). The regression demonstrated an independent risk for ophthalmic morbidity among extremely preterm born offspring (adjusted hazard ratio 3.8, confidence interval 1.6–9.2, $p < 0.01$), as well as very preterm and moderate to late preterm (adjusted hazard ratio 2.2 and 1.5, respectively) as compared with term deliveries. Conclusions: The risk for long-term ophthalmic-related hospitalization of preterm offspring gradually decreases as the gestational age increases.

Keywords: ophthalmic morbidities; retinopathy of prematurity; gestational age; preterm delivery

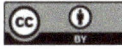

Citation: Tsumi, E.; Hazan, I.; Regev, T.; Leeman, S.; Barrett, C.; Fried Regev, N.; Sheiner, E. The Association between Gestational Age and Risk for Long Term Ophthalmic Morbidities among Offspring Delivered in Different Preterm Subgroups. *J. Clin. Med.* **2022**, *11*, 2562. https://doi.org/10.3390/jcm11092562

Academic Editors: Sylvie Girard and Ferdinando Antonio Gulino

Received: 17 March 2022
Accepted: 29 April 2022
Published: 2 May 2022

Publisher's Note: MDPI stays neutral with regard to jurisdictional claims in published maps and institutional affiliations.

Copyright: © 2022 by the authors. Licensee MDPI, Basel, Switzerland. This article is an open access article distributed under the terms and conditions of the Creative Commons Attribution (CC BY) license (https://creativecommons.org/licenses/by/4.0/).

1. Introduction

The consequences of prematurity are well established in literature, causing long-term and potentially severe effects on pediatric and infantile morbidity and mortality [1,2]. With incomplete maturation, preterm infants are at a greater risk for developing a wide spectrum of medical complications, including hypothermia, jaundice, respiratory disorders [3], immunologic problems [4], neurodevelopmental problems [5–7], increased susceptibility to infections, hypoglycemia and feeding problems. In accordance with preterm newborns' shorter intrauterine periods, ocular development in preterm infants is also subject to a number of abnormal influences, given the reduced time for proper growth and support in a unique environment [8]. Previous literature demonstrated that children who were born very preterm (28–32 weeks) are at a significantly higher risk for abnormal visual and neurological development, when compared to children born at full term [9]. These abnormalities include retinopathy of prematurity (ROP), strabismus, color vision deficits, visual field defects, decreased visual acuity and refractive error [10].

The World Health Organization (WHO) subcategorizes preterm births based on gestational age: extremely preterm (less than 28 weeks delivery), very preterm (28 to 32 weeks delivery), moderate to late preterm (32 to 37 weeks delivery) [11].

A recent study showed that long-term ophthalmic morbidities of offspring is significantly associated with early term delivery [12]. Early preterm-born offspring were found to have an independent risk for long-term ophthalmic morbidity (adjusted hazard ratio 2.51, confidence interval 1.91–3.29) as compared with full term offspring. In our study, we sought to investigate one step further to understand the relative risk for long-term ophthalmic morbidity between the different subcategories of preterm deliveries.

2. Materials and Methods

A retrospective cohort study of all singleton pregnancies in women who gave birth between the years 1991 and 2014 was conducted. Data was taken from the Soroka Univer-sity Medical Center (SUMC), the major tertiary hospital in the Negev region of Israel and the largest birth center in the country. The Negev region has continued to see increasing immigration since the 1990s. Therefore, the present study was based on non-selective population data. The study protocol was a received informed consent exemption by the SUMC institutional review board and was exempt from informed consent. The study population included two different ethnic groups: Jewish and Bedouins, who differ in their economic status, levels of education, and traditional beliefs [13]. However, prenatal care services are available to all Israeli citizens free of charge (covered by universal national health Insurance) [13]. Nevertheless, prenatal care services utilization is lower in Bedouin women as compared to Jewish women for a variety of social, cultural, and geographical access issues [14,15].

The primary exposure was defined as pre-term delivery (before 37 weeks). The control groups consisted of newborns born at later gestations. Gestational age was based on the best obstetric estimate determined by providers and used for clinical decision making. The standard criteria used involved consideration of the clinical history and earliest ultrasound scan. If the last menstrual period (LMP) was certain and consistent with the ultrasound, dating was based on the LMP. If the ultrasound was not consistent with the LMP, or the LMP was unknown, ultrasound data were used to determine gestational age.

Excluded from the study were fetuses with congenital malformations or chromosomal abnormalities, as well as perinatal mortality cases (intrauterine fetal death, intrapartum death, and post-partum death) and nonsingleton births. All offspring were divided into four groups according to their gestational age at delivery: extremely preterm birth: 24–28 gestational weeks, very preterm birth: 28–32 gestational weeks, moderate to late preterm birth: 32–37 gestational weeks and term deliveries: above 37 weeks.

The long-term outcomes assessed included all hospitalizations of offspring at SUMC until the age of 18 years that involved ophthalmic morbidity. The term "ophthalmic morbidity" included four categories: visual disturbances, retinopathy of prematurity, ocular infection and hospitalization. All diagnoses during hospitalization were predefined according to a set of ICD-9 procedures and diagnostic codes, detailed in Table A1.

Follow-up was terminated once any of the following occurred: after the first hospitalization, due to any of the predefined ophthalmic morbidities, any hospitalization resulting in death of the child, or when the child reached 18 years of age (calculated by date of birth).

Data was collected from two databases that were cross-linked and merged: the computerized hospitalization database of SUMC ("Demog-ICD9"), and the computerized perinatal database of the Obstetrics and Gynecology Department. The perinatal database consists of information recorded immediately following an obstetrician delivery. Experienced medical secretaries routinely reviewed the information prior to entering it into the database to ensure maximal completeness and accuracy. Coding was carried out after assessing medical prenatal care records, as well as routine hospital documents.

The SPSS package 23rd ed. (IBM/SPSS, Chicago, IL, USA) was used for statistical analysis. Categorical data is shown in counts and rates. Associations between the gestational age categories, background and outcome characteristics were assessed using the chi-square and ANOVA tests. In order to demonstrate the cumulative hospitalization incidences over time among the study groups, a Kaplan–Meier survival curve was used, and the log-rank test was used to assess the difference between the curves.

For the purposes of establishing an independent association between specific gestational age and the future incidence of ophthalmic-related hospitalizations of the offspring, a Cox regression model was constructed. The model was adjusted for confounding and clinically significant variables, including maternal age and diabetes (pre-gestational and gestational). All analyses were two-sided, and a p-value of ≤ 0.05 was statistically considered.

3. Results

A total of 243,363 deliveries were included in the study; 405 were between 24–28 gestational weeks (0.2%), 1084 deliveries were between 28–32 weeks (0.4%), 14,956 deliveries were between 32–37 weeks (6.1%) and 226,918 occurred at $\geq$37 gestational weeks (93.2%).

Table 1 summarizes maternal characteristics by delivery week category. Maternal age was similar in all delivery groups, with an overall average of 28.08 ± 6.3. Diabetes was more likely to occur in deliveries between 32–37 weeks (7.5%). Hypertensive disorders were more common in deliveries between 28–32 weeks (17.7%).

Table 1. Maternal characteristics according to gestational age.

Maternal Characteristic	Extremely Preterm: 24–28 Weeks (n = 405)	Very Preterm: 28–32 Weeks (n = 1084)	Moderate to Late Preterm: 32–37 Weeks (n = 14,956)	Term Deliveries: more than 37 weeks (n = 22,6918)	p-Value
Ethnicity, n (%) Jewish Bedouin	190 (46.9%) 215 (53.1%)	463 (42.7%) 621 (57.3%)	6883 (46%) 8073 (54%)	107,673 (47.5%) 119,245 (52.5%)	<0.01
Maternal age, years, mean ± SD	28.44 ± 6.5	28.16 ± 6.3	28.14 ± 6.2	28.16 ± 5.7	<0.01
Diabetes [1], n (%)	5 (1.2%)	57 (5.3%)	1118 (7.5%)	10,973 (4.8%)	<0.01
Hypertensive disease [2], n (%)	40 (9.9%)	192 (17.7%)	1839 (12.3%)	10,169 (4.5%)	<0.01

[1] Including pre gestational and gestational diabetes; [2] Including pre gestational, gestational hypertension and pre-eclampsia.

Table 2 summarizes pregnancy outcomes of all four groups. Mean birth weight was positively associated to gestational age; ranging from 855.1 ± 429.5 for 24–28 weeks of age to 3264 ± 446.6 among the mature group, while small for gestational age (SGA) as well as low birth weight (LBW) were most common in the former group (13.3% and 97.5% respectively). Cesarean deliveries were significantly more common among women in 28–32 weeks of gestation (44.8%, p-value < 0.01).

Table 2. Pregnancy outcomes for children (age < 18) by delivery week.

Pregnancy Outcome	Extremely Preterm: 24–28 Weeks (n = 405)	Very Preterm: 28–32 Weeks (n = 1084)	Moderate to Late Preterm: 32–37 Weeks (n = 14,676)	Term Deliveries: more than 37 Weeks (n = 226,917)	p-Value
Birthweight, gr mean ± SD	855.1 ± 429.5	1560.7 ± 623.4	2532.4 ± 506.3	3264.2 ± 446.6	<0.01
Small for gestational age [1], n (%)	54 (13.3%)	54 (5%)	607 (4.1%)	10,547 (4.6%)	<0.01
Low birth weight [2], n (%)	395 (97.5%)	992 (91.5%)	7030 (47%)	7805 (3.4%)	<0.01
Cesarean delivery, n (%)	139 (34.3%)	486 (44.8%)	4444 (29.7%)	27,908 (12.3%)	<0.01

[1] Small for gestational age (SGA) < 5th percentile for gestational age; [2] Low birth weight (LBW) < 2500 g.

The long-term ophthalmological morbidities based on hospitalizations is presented in Table 3. Rates of visual disturbances and retinopathy of prematurity (ROP) were significantly higher among the 24–28 gestational weeks group (0.7%, p-value < 0.01; 1.4%, p-value < 0.01 respectively), while ocular infection was highest among newborns in the 28–32 weeks of gestation (0.9%, p-value < 0.01). Total ophthalmic hospitalization rates were highest among the 24–28 gestational weeks group (3.6%, p-value < 0.01 using the chi-square test for trends), and gradually decreased with increasing gestational week (2% among 28–32 weeks, 1.4% among 32–37 weeks, and 0.9% among 37+ weeks). A decrease in the number of hospitalizations with gestational age was also documented while stratifying for ethnicity. Offspring born between 24–28 weeks had the highest cumulative incidence of hospitalizations (Figure 1) due to ophthalmological morbidity, followed by offspring born at 28–36 and those born at $\geq$37 gestational weeks ($p < 0.001$).

Table 3. Selected long-term ophthalmological morbidities for children (age < 18) by delivery week.

Ophthalmological Morbidity		Extremely Preterm: 24–28 Weeks (n = 138)	Very Preterm: 28–32 Weeks (n = 891)	Moderate to Late Preterm: 32–37 Weeks (n = 14,676)	Term Deliveries: more than 37 Weeks (n = 226,482)	p-Value
Visual disturbances, n (%)		1 (0.7%)	0 (0%)	36 (0.2%)	245 (0.1%)	<0.01
ROP, n (%)		2 (1.4%)	2 (0.2%)	0 (0%)	0 (0%)	<0.01
Ocular Infections, n (%)		1 (0.7%)	8 (0.9%)	123 (0.8%)	1336 (0.6%)	0.02
Total ophthalmic Hospitalization, n (%)	Bedouin	2 (1.4%)	12 (1.3%)	123 (0.8%)	1190 (0.5%)	<0.01
	Jewish	3 (2.2%)	6 (0.7%)	85 (0.6%)	907 (0.4%)	<0.01
	All	5 (3.6%)	18 (2%)	208 (1.4%)	2097 (0.9%)	<0.01

In the multivariate Cox regression model for offspring long-term risk of ophthalmic-related hospitalizations (Table 4), earlier deliveries were associated with higher risk for hospitalization, compared to the most mature group (24–28) weeks: HR = 3.8; CI95% 2.6–9.2; 28–32 weeks: HR = 2.2; CI95% 1.4–3.5; 32–37 weeks: HR = 1.5; CI95% 1.3–1.7).

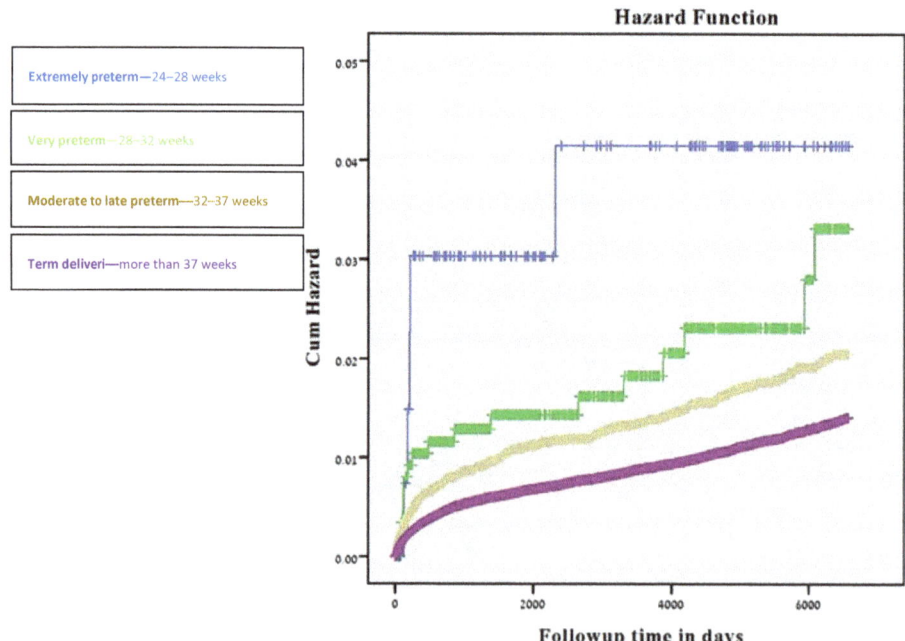

Figure 1. Kaplan-Meier survival curve demonstrating the cumulative incidence of. ophthalmological-related hospitalizations compared to delivery time in weeks.

Table 4. Cox regression analysis of the association between week of birth and ophthalmic-related hospitalization of children (age < 18).

	Hazard Ratio	95% CI	p-Value
Extremely preterm: 24–28 weeks	3.8	1.6–9.2	<0.01
Very preterm: 28–32 weeks	2.2	1.4–3.5	<0.01
Moderate to late preterm: 32–37 weeks	1.5	1.3–1.7	<0.01
Term deliveries: more than 37 weeks	1 (Reference)		
Mother age at birth	0.9	0.98–0.99	0.02
Diabetes	1.0	0.8–1.2	0.6

4. Discussion

This large population-based cohort study demonstrates an increased risk for childhood and adolescence long-term ophthalmic morbidities as the gestational age becomes earlier among the pre-term deliveries. The risk remained significantly elevated among all the preterm groups while controlling for relevant maternal factors.

Numerous studies have identified an association between early gestational age at birth and the risk of poor health outcomes, based on incidence of morbidities, mortality and hospitalization rates [16,17]. A growing body of evidence has also shown ophthalmic morbidity among preterm infants. Kozeis et al. [18] found preterm infants to be associated with impairment of some aspects of visual function.

Although the pathophysiology is still not fully understood, complex multifactorial mechanisms have been suggested as the potential causes for ocular damage from preterm delivery. The suggested mechanisms include deficiencies in both innate and adaptive immunity [19], hypoxic-ischemic induced inflammation and cytokine injury, reperfusion injury, toxin-mediated injury, infection [20,21], and insufficient endogenous hormones (e.g., Cortisol & thyroxin), often exhibited as transient hypothyroxinemia of prematurity (THOP) [22].

Vast epidemiological studies conducted worldwide on ROP showed that despite geographical variability, the incidence of ROP was similar [14–18]. A study conducted by the Australian and New Zealand Neonatal Network (ANZNN) showed that the incidence of severe ROP was higher (34%) in infants born before 25 weeks gestation when compared to infants born at 25–26 weeks gestation (12.9%) [23]. Similar results have been found in North America, the UK and Indonesia [24–26].

Our findings revealed that the highest rate of ROP was observed in infants born at 24–28 weeks gestation (1.4%), with a declining rate for more advanced gestational age and reaching zero cases in those born after 32 weeks' gestation. These results are consistent with previous studies examining the rate of ROP [27–30] and are likely to be explained by the fact that ROP is a disease of developing blood vessels, which are still considered underdeveloped at the beginning of the third trimester [31].

Additional long-term ophthalmological morbidities, such as visual disturbances, were examined in our study and showed the same pattern. The higher visual disturbances in preterm babies are a consequence of the higher retinopathy rate and other reasons e.g., osteopenia of prematurity [32]. Other types of vision disturbances include sub-categories, such as strabismus (both exotropia and esotropia), refractive errors, visual field deficits, color vision errors, astigmatism, cortical blindness and more. A recent study comparing strabismus in premature and term children found that the risk for strabismus in premature children was substantially higher than in full-term children (16.2% vs. 3.2%) [33]. Other ophthalmological morbidities related to prematurity, such as ROP, were linked to increased risk for strabismus as well [34].

Many factors contribute to the increased susceptibility of preterm infants to infections. Prematurity is associated with underdeveloped ocular surface defense mechanisms and has also been associated with neonatal conjunctivitis [35]. While previous studies showed an increase in the risk for general ocular infection among preterm newborns compared to term newborns [36], our analysis did not show a conclusive trend. Infants born between 24–28 weeks of gestation showed a lower proportion of ocular infections compared to those born during weeks 28–32 (0.7% compared to 0.9% respectively). This result could be explained by the smaller size of the preterm group and requires further analysis.

The key strength of our study was the use of a large cohort in a single medical center providing broad follow-up of children up to 18 years of age. This allowed for the investigation of substantially larger numbers of infants to be followed-up on than could be achieved by individual NICU follow-up studies, and simplified the monitoring of all infants for the purposes of comparison.

A major limitation of our study is its retrospective nature, as such studies may only suggest an association rather than causation. An additional limitation is the fact that information on other important risk factors, such as lifestyle, nutrition, perinatal treatment and other family factors was not available in the datasets. Two more challenges stemmed from the choice of ophthalmic-related hospitalizations as the present study's endpoint: (1) Most of the ophthalmic morbidity is probably catered to in an outpatient setting (as discussed earlier). However, all significant ocular morbidity is routed to the SUMC, as it is the only tertiary hospital in the South of Israel (2) Offspring born earlier are more likely to be hospitalized in general, and therefore may be more frequently diagnosed with ophthalmic morbidities.

5. Conclusions

Our study was able to find a significant association between degree of prematurity and long-term ocular morbidities up to 18 years of age. A markedly increasing risk of severe adverse neonatal outcomes was observed as gestational age decreased. Further studies could raise awareness for early interventions, improve children's health outcomes and decrease the burden on health care systems attributed to these diseases.

Author Contributions: Conceptualization, I.H. and E.S.; Formal analysis, E.S.; Methodology, E.T., C.B. and E.S.; Project administration, E.T.; Resources, E.T. and T.R.; Supervision, I.H.; Validation, E.T., N.F.R. and E.S.; Writing—original draft, I.H.; Writing—review & editing, I.H., S.L. and E.S. All authors have read and agreed to the published version of the manuscript.

Funding: This research received no external funding.

Institutional Review Board Statement: The study was conducted in accordance with the Declaration of Helsinki, and approved by the Institutional Review Board of Soroka University Medical Center (protocol #0357-19-SOR, October 2019).

Informed Consent Statement: Patient consent was waived since the analysis was based on a deidentified computerized database.

Data Availability Statement: Unavailable according to the Helsinki protocol.

Conflicts of Interest: The authors declare no conflict of interest.

Appendix A

Table A1. Supplement Data—Ophthalmic Diagnoses.

Group	Subgroup	Code	Diagnosis Description
Ophthalmic	Infectious inflammatory	370	KERATITIS
		3643	UNSPECIFIED IRIDOCYCLITIS
		3708	OTHER FORMS OF KERATITIS
		3709	UNSPECIFIED KERATITIS
		3720	ACUTE CONJUNCTIVITIS

Table A1. Cont.

Group	Subgroup	Code	Diagnosis Description
		3723	OTHER AND UNSPECIFIED CONJUNCTIVITIS
		3729	UNSPECIFIED DISORDER OF CONJUNCTIVA
		3732	CHALAZION
		3736	PARASITIC INFESTATION OF EYELID
		3739	UNSPECIFIED INFLAMMATION OF EYELID
		36000	PURULENT ENDOPHTHALMITIS, UNSPECIFIED
		36011	SYMPATHETIC UVEITIS
		36012	PANUVEITIS
		36019	OTHER ENDOPHTHALMITIS
		36212	EXUDATIVE RETINOPATHY
		36320	CHORIORETINITIS, UNSPECIFIED
		36322	HARADA'S DISEASE
		36403	SECONDARY IRIDOCYCLITIS, INFECTIOUS
		36404	SECONDARY IRIDOCYCLITIS, NONINFECTIOUS
		36410	CHRONIC IRIDOCYCLITIS, UNSPECIFIED
		36424	VOGT-KOYANAGI SYNDROME
		37021	PUNCTATE KERATITIS
		37031	PHLYCTENULAR KERATOCONJUNCTIVITIS
		37040	KERATOCONJUNCTIVITIS, UNSPECIFIED
		37049	OTHER KERATOCONJUNCTIVITIS
		37055	CORNEAL ABSCESS
		37059	OTHER INTERSTITIAL AND DEEP KERATITIS
		37200	ACUTE CONJUNCTIVITIS, UNSPECIFIED
		37202	ACUTE FOLLICULAR CONJUNCTIVITIS
		37203	OTHER MUCOPURULENT CONJUNCTIVITIS
		37205	ACUTE ATOPIC CONJUNCTIVITIS
		37211	SIMPLE CHRONIC CONJUNCTIVITIS
		37213	VERNAL CONJUNCTIVITIS
		37214	OTHER CHRONIC ALLERGIC CONJUNCTIVITIS
		37220	BLEPHAROCONJUNCTIVITIS, UNSPECIFIED
		37230	CONJUNCTIVITIS, UNSPECIFIED
		37240	PTERYGIUM, UNSPECIFIED
		37261	GRANULOMA OF CONJUNCTIVA
		37300	BLEPHARITIS, UNSPECIFIED
		37311	HORDEOLUM EXTERNUM
		37312	HORDEOLUM INTERNUM
		37313	ABSCESS OF EYELID
		37400	ENTROPION, UNSPECIFIED
		37405	TRICHIASIS OF EYELID WITHOUT ENTROPION
		37500	DACRYOADENITIS, UNSPECIFIED
		37502	CHRONIC DACRYOADENITIS
		37530	DACRYOCYSTITIS, UNSPECIFIED
		37532	ACUTE DACRYOCYSTITIS
		37541	CHRONIC CANALICULITIS
		37542	CHRONIC DACRYOCYSTITIS
		37543	LACRIMAL MUCOCELE

Table A1. *Cont.*

Group	Subgroup	Code	Diagnosis Description
		37600	ACUTE INFLAMMATION OF ORBIT, UNSPECIFIED
		37601	ORBITAL CELLULITIS
		37610	CHRONIC INFLAMMATION OF ORBIT, UNSPECIFIED
		37611	ORBITAL GRANULOMA
		37612	ORBITAL MYOSITIS
		37613	PARASITIC INFESTATION OF ORBIT
		37730	OPTIC NEURITIS, UNSPECIFIED
		37731	OPTIC PAPILLITIS
		37732	RETROBULBAR NEURITIS (ACUTE)
		37739	OTHER OPTIC NEURITIS
		37900	SCLERITIS, UNSPECIFIED
		37909	OTHER SCLERITIS
		376010	PERIORBITAL CELLULITIS
	Retinopathy of prematurity	36220	RETINOPATHY OF PREMATURITY, UNSPECIFIED
		36221	RETROLENTAL FIBROPLASIA
		36223	RETINOPATHY OF PREMATURITY, STAGE 1
		362211	RETINOPATHY OF PREMATURITY
	Visual disturbances	3670	HYPERMETROPIA
		3671	MYOPIA
		3672	ASTIGMATISM
		3682	DIPLOPIA
		3688	OTHER SPECIFIED VISUAL DISTURBANCES
		3689	UNSPECIFIED VISUAL DISTURBANCE
		3698	UNQUALIFIED VISUAL LOSS, ONE EYE
		3699	UNSPECIFIED VISUAL LOSS
		3780	ESOTROPIA
		36021	PROGRESSIVE HIGH (DEGENERATIVE) MYOPIA
		36720	ASTIGMATISM, UNSPECIFIED
		36731	ANISOMETROPIA
		36781	TRANSIENT REFRACTIVE CHANGE
		36800	AMBLYOPIA, UNSPECIFIED
		36801	STRABISMIC AMBLYOPIA
		36811	SUDDEN VISUAL LOSS
		36812	TRANSIENT VISUAL LOSS
		36840	VISUAL FIELD DEFECT, UNSPECIFIED
		36900	BLINDNESS OF BOTH EYES, IMPAIRMENT LEVEL NOT FURTHER SPECIFIED
		36960	BLINDNESS, ONE EYE, NOT OTHERWISE SPECIFIED
		36970	LOW VISION, ONE EYE, NOT OTHERWISE SPECIFIED
		37775	CORTICAL BLINDNESS
		37800	ESOTROPIA, UNSPECIFIED
		37801	MONOCULAR ESOTROPIA
		37805	ALTERNATING ESOTROPIA
		37810	EXOTROPIA, UNSPECIFIED
		37815	ALTERNATING EXOTROPIA

Table A1. Cont.

Group	Subgroup	Code	Diagnosis Description
		37817	ALTERNATING EXOTROPIA WITH V PATTERN
		37820	INTERMITTENT HETEROTROPIA, UNSPECIFIED
		37821	INTERMITTENT ESOTROPIA, MONOCULAR
		37824	INTERMITTENT EXOTROPIA, ALTERNATING
		37830	HETEROTROPIA, UNSPECIFIED
		37831	HYPERTROPIA
		37832	HYPOTROPIA
		37835	ACCOMMODATIVE COMPONENT IN ESOTROPIA
		37881	PALSY OF CONJUGATE GAZE
		37885	ANOMALIES OF DIVERGENCE
	Not otherwise specified	3612	SEROUS RETINAL DETACHMENT
		3619	UNSPECIFIED RETINAL DETACHMENT
		3633	CHORIORETINAL SCARS
		3648	OTHER DISORDERS OF IRIS AND CILIARY BODY
		3651	OPEN-ANGLE GLAUCOMA
		3659	UNSPECIFIED GLAUCOMA
		3669	UNSPECIFIED CATARACT
		3769	UNSPECIFIED DISORDER OF ORBIT
		3770	PAPILLEDEMA
		3789	UNSPECIFIED DISORDER OF EYE MOVEMENTS
		3798	OTHER SPECIFIED DISORDERS OF EYE AND ADNEXA
		36020	DEGENERATIVE DISORDER OF GLOBE, UNSPECIFIED
		36023	SIDEROSIS OF GLOBE
		36030	HYPOTONY OF EYE, UNSPECIFIED
		36033	HYPOTONY ASSOCIATED WITH OTHER OCULAR DISORDERS
		36041	BLIND HYPOTENSIVE EYE
		36043	HEMOPHTHALMOS, EXCEPT CURRENT INJURY
		36044	LEUCOCORIA
		36100	RETINAL DETACHMENT WITH RETINAL DEFECT, UNSPECIFIED
		36103	RECENT RETINAL DETACHMENT, PARTIAL, WITH GIANT TEAR
		36104	RECENT RETINAL DETACHMENT, PARTIAL, WITH RETINAL DIALYSIS
		36105	RECENT RETINAL DETACHMENT, TOTAL OR SUBTOTAL
		36107	OLD RETINAL DETACHMENT, TOTAL OR SUBTOTAL
		36110	RETINOSCHISIS, UNSPECIFIED
		36133	MULTIPLE DEFECTS OF RETINA WITHOUT DETACHMENT
		36181	TRACTION DETACHMENT OF RETINA
		36202	PROLIFERATIVE DIABETIC RETINOPATHY
		36210	BACKGROUND RETINOPATHY, UNSPECIFIED
		36211	HYPERTENSIVE RETINOPATHY
		36216	RETINAL NEOVASCULARIZATION NOS
		36229	OTHER NONDIABETIC PROLIFERATIVE RETINOPATHY
		36231	CENTRAL RETINAL ARTERY OCCLUSION

Table A1. Cont.

Group	Subgroup	Code	Diagnosis Description
		36234	TRANSIENT RETINAL ARTERIAL OCCLUSION
		36235	CENTRAL RETINAL VEIN OCCLUSION
		36240	RETINAL LAYER SEPARATION, UNSPECIFIED
		36250	MACULAR DEGENERATION (SENILE) OF RETINA, UNSPECIFIED
		36254	MACULAR CYST, HOLE, OR PSEUDOHOLE OF RETINA
		36256	MACULAR PUCKERING OF RETINA
		36263	LATTICE DEGENERATION OF RETINA
		36270	HEREDITARY RETINAL DYSTROPHY, UNSPECIFIED
		36273	VITREORETINAL DYSTROPHIES
		36274	PIGMENTARY RETINAL DYSTROPHY
		36281	RETINAL HEMORRHAGE
		36330	CHORIORETINAL SCAR, UNSPECIFIED
		36332	OTHER MACULAR SCARS OF RETINA
		36361	CHOROIDAL HEMORRHAGE, UNSPECIFIED
		36370	CHOROIDAL DETACHMENT, UNSPECIFIED
		36372	HEMORRHAGIC CHOROIDAL DETACHMENT
		36405	HYPOPYON
		36441	HYPHEMA OF IRIS AND CILIARY BODY
		36470	ADHESIONS OF IRIS, UNSPECIFIED
		36471	POSTERIOR SYNECHIAE OF IRIS
		36472	ANTERIOR SYNECHIAE OF IRIS
		36474	ADHESIONS AND DISRUPTIONS OF PUPILLARY MEMBRANES
		36475	PUPILLARY ABNORMALITIES
		36476	IRIDODIALYSIS
		36477	RECESSION OF CHAMBER ANGLE OF EYE
		36489	OTHER DISORDERS OF IRIS AND CILIARY BODY
		36500	PREGLAUCOMA, UNSPECIFIED
		36504	OCULAR HYPERTENSION
		36514	GLAUCOMA OF CHILDHOOD
		36520	PRIMARY ANGLE-CLOSURE GLAUCOMA, UNSPECIFIED
		36560	GLAUCOMA ASSOCIATED WITH UNSPECIFIED OCULAR DISORDER
		36600	NONSENILE CATARACT, UNSPECIFIED
		36610	SENILE CATARACT, UNSPECIFIED
		36612	INCIPIENT SENILE CATARACT
		36616	SENILE NUCLEAR SCLEROSIS
		36620	TRAUMATIC CATARACT, UNSPECIFIED
		36630	CATARACTA COMPLICATA, UNSPECIFIED
		36650	AFTER-CATARACT, UNSPECIFIED
		36813	VISUAL DISCOMFORT
		36815	OTHER VISUAL DISTORTIONS AND ENTOPTIC PHENOMENA
		36816	PSYCHOPHYSICAL VISUAL DISTURBANCES
		37000	CORNEAL ULCER, UNSPECIFIED
		37003	CENTRAL CORNEAL ULCER
		37004	HYPOPYON ULCER

Table A1. Cont.

Group	Subgroup	Code	Diagnosis Description
		37100	CORNEAL OPACITY, UNSPECIFIED
		37105	PHTHISICAL CORNEA
		37120	CORNEAL EDEMA, UNSPECIFIED
		37123	BULLOUS KERATOPATHY
		37140	CORNEAL DEGENERATION, UNSPECIFIED
		37142	RECURRENT EROSION OF CORNEA
		37143	BAND-SHAPED KERATOPATHY
		37150	HEREDITARY CORNEAL DYSTROPHY, UNSPECIFIED
		37157	ENDOTHELIAL CORNEAL DYSTROPHY
		37158	OTHER POSTERIOR CORNEAL DYSTROPHIES
		37160	KERATOCONUS, UNSPECIFIED
		37162	KERATOCONUS, ACUTE HYDROPS
		37170	CORNEAL DEFORMITY, UNSPECIFIED
		37172	DESCEMETOCELE
		37263	SYMBLEPHARON
		37272	CONJUNCTIVAL HEMORRHAGE
		37273	CONJUNCTIVAL EDEMA
		37274	VASCULAR ABNORMALITIES OF CONJUNCTIVA
		37275	CONJUNCTIVAL CYSTS
		37289	OTHER DISORDERS OF CONJUNCTIVA
		37420	LAGOPHTHALMOS, UNSPECIFIED
		37430	PTOSIS OF EYELID, UNSPECIFIED
		37451	XANTHELASMA OF EYELID
		37482	EDEMA OF EYELID
		37484	CYSTS OF EYELIDS
		37489	OTHER DISORDERS OF EYELID
		37515	TEAR FILM INSUFFICIENCY, UNSPECIFIED
		37520	EPIPHORA, UNSPECIFIED AS TO CAUSE
		37521	EPIPHORA DUE TO EXCESS LACRIMATION
		37552	STENOSIS OF LACRIMAL PUNCTUM
		37553	STENOSIS OF LACRIMAL CANALICULI
		37554	STENOSIS OF LACRIMAL SAC
		37555	OBSTRUCTION OF NASOLACRIMAL DUCT, NEONATAL
		37556	STENOSIS OF NASOLACRIMAL DUCT, ACQUIRED
		37561	LACRIMAL FISTULA
		37630	EXOPHTHALMOS, UNSPECIFIED
		37633	ORBITAL EDEMA OR CONGESTION
		37641	HYPERTELORISM OF ORBIT
		37646	ENLARGEMENT OF ORBIT
		37651	ENOPHTHALMOS DUE TO ATROPHY OF ORBITAL TISSUE
		37681	ORBITAL CYSTS
		37689	OTHER ORBITAL DISORDERS
		37700	PAPILLEDEMA, UNSPECIFIED
		37703	PAPILLEDEMA ASSOCIATED WITH RETINAL DISORDER
		37710	OPTIC ATROPHY, UNSPECIFIED

Table A1. *Cont.*

Group	Subgroup	Code	Diagnosis Description
		37721	DRUSEN OF OPTIC DISC
		37724	PSEUDOPAPILLEDEMA
		37741	ISCHEMIC OPTIC NEUROPATHY
		37749	OTHER DISORDERS OF OPTIC NERVE
		37852	THIRD OR OCULOMOTOR NERVE PALSY, TOTAL
		37853	FOURTH OR TROCHLEAR NERVE PALSY
		37854	SIXTH OR ABDUCENS NERVE PALSY
		37855	EXTERNAL OPHTHALMOPLEGIA
		37871	DUANE'S SYNDROME
		37887	OTHER DISSOCIATED DEVIATION OF EYE MOVEMENTS
		37923	VITREOUS HEMORRHAGE
		37924	OTHER VITREOUS OPACITIES
		37929	OTHER DISORDERS OF VITREOUS
		37931	APHAKIA
		37932	SUBLUXATION OF LENS
		37933	ANTERIOR DISLOCATION OF LENS
		37934	POSTERIOR DISLOCATION OF LENS
		37941	ANISOCORIA
		37942	MIOSIS (PERSISTENT), NOT DUE TO MIOTICS
		37943	MYDRIASIS (PERSISTENT), NOT DUE TO MYDRIATICS
		37950	NYSTAGMUS, UNSPECIFIED
		37951	CONGENITAL NYSTAGMUS
		37952	LATENT NYSTAGMUS
		37954	NYSTAGMUS ASSOCIATED WITH DISORDERS OF THE VESTIBULAR SYSTEM
		37955	DISSOCIATED NYSTAGMUS
		37956	OTHER FORMS OF NYSTAGMUS
		37959	OTHER IRREGULARITIES OF EYE MOVEMENTS
		37991	PAIN IN OR AROUND EYE
		37992	SWELLING OR MASS OF EYE
		37993	REDNESS OR DISCHARGE OF EYE
		37999	OTHER ILL-DEFINED DISORDERS OF EYEa

References

1. Newman, D.E.; Paamoni-Keren, O.; Press, F.; Wiznitzer, A.; Mazor, M.; Sheiner, E. Neonatal outcome in preterm deliveries between 23 and 27 weeks' gestation with and without preterm premature rupture of membranes. *Arch. Gynecol. Obstet.* **2009**, *280*, 7–11. [CrossRef]
2. Vohr, B. Long-term outcomes of moderately preterm, late preterm, and early term infants. *Clin. Perinatol.* **2013**, *40*, 739–751. [CrossRef]
3. Gutvirtz, G.; Wainstock, T.; Sheiner, E.; Pariente, G. Prematurity and Long-Term Respiratory Morbidity—What Is the Critical Gestational Age Threshold? *J. Clin. Med.* **2022**, *11*, 751. [CrossRef]
4. Davidesko, S.; Wainstock, T.; Sheiner, E.; Pariente, G. Long-Term Infectious Morbidity of Premature Infants: Is There a Critical Threshold? *J. Clin. Med.* **2020**, *9*, 3008. [CrossRef]
5. Zer, S.; Wainstock, T.; Sheiner, E.; Miodownik, S.; Pariente, G. Identifying the Critical Threshold for Long-Term Pediatric Neurological Hospitalizations of the Offspring in Preterm Delivery. *J. Clin. Med.* **2021**, *10*, 2919. [CrossRef]
6. Torchin, H.; Morgan, A.S.; Ancel, P.-Y. International comparisons of neurodevelopmental outcomes in infants born very preterm. *Semin. Fetal. Neonatal Med.* **2020**, *25*, 101109. [CrossRef]
7. Rogers, E.E.; Hintz, S.R. Early neurodevelopmental outcomes of extremely preterm infants. *Semin. Perinatol.* **2016**, *40*, 497–509. [CrossRef]

8. O'Connor, A.R.; Wilson, C.M.; Fielder, A.R. Ophthalmological problems associated with preterm birth. *Eye* **2007**, *21*, 1254–1260. [CrossRef]
9. Leung, M.P.; Thompson, B.; Black, J.; Dai, S.; Alsweiler, J.M. The effects of preterm birth on visual development. *Clin. Exp. Optom.* **2018**, *101*, 4–12. [CrossRef]
10. Allen, M.C.; Cristofalo, E.A.; Kim, C. Outcomes of Preterm Infants: Morbidity Replaces Mortality. *Clin. Perinatol.* **2011**, *38*, 441–454. [CrossRef]
11. Preterm Birth. Available online: https://www.who.int/news-room/fact-sheets/detail/preterm-birth (accessed on 16 November 2021).
12. Ben-Shmuel, A.; Sheiner, E.; Tsumi, E.; Wainstock, T.; Feinblum, D.; Walfisch, A. Early-term deliveries and long-term pediatric ophthalmic morbidity of the offspring. *Int. J. Gynaecol. Obstet. Off. Organ Int. Fed. Gynaecol. Obstet.* **2021**, 1–7. [CrossRef] [PubMed]
13. Sheiner, E.; Hallak, M.; Twizer, I.; Mazor, M.; Katz, M.; Shoham-Vardi, I. Lack of prenatal care in two different societies living in the same region and sharing the same medical facilities. *J. Obstet. Gynaecol. J. Inst. Obstet. Gynaecol.* **2001**, *21*, 453–458. [CrossRef] [PubMed]
14. Estis-Deaton, A.; Sheiner, E.; Wainstock, T.; Landau, D.; Walfisch, A. The association between inadequate prenatal care and future healthcare use among offspring in the Bedouin population. *Int. J. Gynaecol. Obstet. Off. Organ Int. Fed. Gynaecol. Obstet.* **2017**, *139*, 284–289. [CrossRef] [PubMed]
15. Abu-Ghanem, S.; Sheiner, E.; Sherf, M.; Wiznitzer, A.; Sergienko, R.; Shoham-Vardi, I. Lack of prenatal care in a traditional community: Trends and perinatal outcomes. *Arch. Gynecol. Obstet.* **2012**, *285*, 1237–1242. [CrossRef]
16. Stephens, A.S.; Lain, S.J.; Roberts, C.L.; Bowen, J.R.; Nassar, N. Survival, Hospitalization, and Acute-Care Costs of Very and Moderate Preterm Infants in the First 6 Years of Life: A Population-Based Study. *J. Pediatr.* **2016**, *169*, 61–68.e3. [CrossRef]
17. Lui, K.; Vento, M.; Modi, N.; Kusuda, S.; Lehtonen, L.; Håkansson, S.; Rusconi, F.; Bassler, D.; Reichman, B.; Yang, J.; et al. Inter-center variability in neonatal outcomes of preterm infants: A longitudinal evaluation of 298 neonatal units in 11 countries. *Semin. Fetal. Neonatal Med.* **2021**, *26*, 101196. [CrossRef]
18. Kozeis, N.; Mavromichali, M.; Soubasi-Griva, V.; Agakidou, E.; Zafiriou, D.; Drossou, V. Visual Function in Preterm Infants without Major Retinopathy of Prematurity or Neurological Complications. *Am. J. Perinatol.* **2012**, *29*, 747–754. [CrossRef]
19. Melville, J.M.; Moss, T.J.M. The immune consequences of preterm birth. *Front. Neurosci.* **2013**, *7*, 79. [CrossRef]
20. Hagberg, H.; Mallard, C.; Jacobsson, B. Role of cytokines in preterm labour and brain injury. *BJOG Int. J. Obstet. Gynaecol.* **2005**, *112* (Suppl. S1), 16–18. [CrossRef]
21. McAdams, R.M.; Juul, S.E. The Role of Cytokines and Inflammatory Cells in Perinatal Brain Injury. *Neurol. Res. Int.* **2012**, *2012*, 1–15. [CrossRef]
22. Rovet, J.; Simic, N. The Role of Transient Hypothyroxinemia of Prematurity in Development of Visual Abilities. *Semin. Perinatol.* **2008**, *32*, 431–437. [CrossRef] [PubMed]
23. Darlow, B.A.; Hutchinson, J.L.; Henderson-Smart, D.J.; Donoghue, D.A.; Simpson, J.M.; Evans, N.J.; Australian and New Zealand Neonatal Network. Prenatal risk factors for severe retinopathy of prematurity in very preterm infants of the Australian and New Zealand Neonatal Network. *Pediatrics* **2005**, *115*, 990–996. [CrossRef] [PubMed]
24. Haines, L. UK population based study of severe retinopathy of prematurity: Screening, treatment, and outcome. *Arch. Dis. Child. Fetal Neonatal Ed.* **2005**, *90*, F240–F244. [CrossRef] [PubMed]
25. Chiang, M.F.; Arons, R.R.; Flynn, J.T.; Starren, J.B. Incidence of retinopathy of prematurity from 1996 to 2000: Analysis of a comprehensive New York state patient database. *Ophthalmology* **2004**, *111*, 1317–1325. [CrossRef] [PubMed]
26. Edy Siswanto, J.; Sauer, P.J. Retinopathy of prematurity in Indonesia: Incidence and risk factors. *J. Neonatal-Perinat. Med.* **2017**, *10*, 85–90. [CrossRef] [PubMed]
27. Chiang, M.-C.; Tang, J.-R.; Yau, K.-I.T.; Yang, C.-M. A proposal of screening guideline for retinopathy of prematurity in Taiwan. *Acta Paediatr. Taiwanica Taiwan Er Ke Yi Xue Hui Za Zhi* **2002**, *43*, 204–207.
28. Ells, A.; Hicks, M.; Fielden, M.; Ingram, A. Severe retinopathy of prematurity: Longitudinal observation of disease and screening implications. *Eye* **2005**, *19*, 138–144. [CrossRef]
29. Reynolds, J.D. Evidence-Based Screening Criteria for Retinopathy of Prematurity: Natural History Data From the CRYO-ROP and LIGHT-ROP Studies. *Arch. Ophthalmol.* **2002**, *120*, 1470. [CrossRef]
30. Wright, K.; Anderson, M.E.; Walker, E.; Lorch, V. Should Fewer Premature Infants Be Screened for Retinopathy of Prematurity in the Managed Care Era? *Pediatrics* **1998**, *102*, 31–34. [CrossRef]
31. Todd, D.A.; Wright, A.; Smith, J.; NICUS Group. Severe retinopathy of prematurity in infants <30 weeks' gestation in New South Wales and the Australian Capital Territory from 1992 to 2002. *Arch. Dis. Child. Fetal Neonatal Ed.* **2007**, *92*, F251–F254. [CrossRef]
32. Pohlandt, F. Hypothesis: Myopia of prematurity is caused by postnatal bone mineral deficiency. *Eur. J. Pediatr.* **1994**, *153*, 234–236. [CrossRef] [PubMed]
33. Holmström, G.; Rydberg, A.; Larsson, E. Prevalence and development of strabismus in 10-year-old premature children: A population-based study. *J. Pediatr. Ophthalmol. Strabismus* **2006**, *43*, 346–352. [CrossRef] [PubMed]
34. Bremer, D.L. Strabismus in Premature Infants in the First Year of Life. *Arch. Ophthalmol.* **1998**, *116*, 329. [CrossRef] [PubMed]

35. Dogru, M.; Karakaya, H.; Baykara, M.; Özmen, A.; Koksal, N.; Goto, E.; Matsumoto, Y.; Kojima, T.; Shimazaki, J.; Tsubota, K. Tear function and ocular surface findings in premature and term babies. *Ophthalmology* **2004**, *111*, 901–905. [CrossRef] [PubMed]
36. Gichuhi, S.; Bosire, R.; Mbori-Ngacha, D.; Gichuhi, C.; Wamalwa, D.; Maleche-Obimbo, E.; Farquhar, C.; Wariua, G.; Otieno, P.; John-Stewart, G.C. Risk factors for neonatal conjunctivitis in babies of HIV-1 infected mothers. *Ophthalmic Epidemiol.* **2009**, *16*, 337–345. [CrossRef] [PubMed]

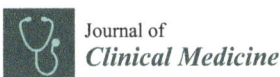

Article

Low Five-Minute Apgar Score and Neurological Morbidities: Does Prematurity Modify the Association?

Tamar Wainstock [1,*] and Eyal Sheiner [2]

[1] Department of Public Health, Faculty of Health Sciences, Ben-Gurion University of the Negev, Beer-Sheva 84417, Israel
[2] Department of Obstetrics and Gynecology, Soroka University Medical Center, Ben-Gurion University of the Negev, Beer-Sheva 84417, Israel; sheiner@bgu.ac.il
* Correspondence: wainstoc@bgu.ac.il; Tel.: +972-5-2311-4880

Abstract: (1) Background: We aimed to study whether a low 5 min Apgar score is associated with pediatric neurological morbidities throughout childhood. (2) Methods: A population-based retrospective cohort study was conducted. The exposed group was defined as offspring with a 5 min Apgar score <7, and the remaining offspring served as the comparison group. The primary outcome was defined as pediatric hospitalizations with any neurological morbidity. Multivariable survival models were used to evaluate the association between the exposure and outcome while adjusting for potential confounders. Additional models were used to study this association separately among term- and preterm-born offspring. (3) Results: The study population included 349,385 singletons born between the years 1991 and 2021, 0.6% (n = 2030) of whom had a 5 min Apgar score <7 (exposed). The cohort was followed for up to 18 years (median ~ 10.6). The incidence of neurological morbidity-related hospitalizations was higher among the exposed group versus the unexposed group (11.3% versus 7.5%, hazard ratio = 1.84; 95%CI 1.58–2.13). A low 5 min Apgar score remained a significant risk factor for neurological hospitalizations after adjusting for preterm delivery, maternal age, hypertension during pregnancy, gestational diabetes mellitus, chorioamnionitis, and delivery mode (adjusted hazard ratio = 1.61; 95%CI 1.39–1.87). However, after modeling term and preterm offspring separately, a low 5 min Apgar score was independently associated with neurological hospitalizations only among offspring born at term (adjusted hazard ratio = 1.16; 95%CI 0.87–1.55 and 1.70; 95%CI 1.42–2.02 for preterm and term offspring, respectively). (4) Conclusions: A low 5 min Apgar score is independently associated with childhood neurological morbidity, specifically among term-born offspring. Although not designed to identify risk for long-term health complications, Apgar scores may be a marker of risk for short- and long-term neurological morbidities among term newborns.

Keywords: Apgar score; neurological morbidities; long-term follow-up; population-based study; retrospective cohort

Citation: Wainstock, T.; Sheiner, E. Low Five-Minute Apgar Score and Neurological Morbidities: Does Prematurity Modify the Association? *J. Clin. Med.* **2022**, *11*, 1922. https://doi.org/10.3390/jcm11071922

Academic Editor: Johannes Ott

Received: 25 February 2022
Accepted: 28 March 2022
Published: 30 March 2022

Publisher's Note: MDPI stays neutral with regard to jurisdictional claims in published maps and institutional affiliations.

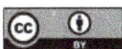

Copyright: © 2022 by the authors. Licensee MDPI, Basel, Switzerland. This article is an open access article distributed under the terms and conditions of the Creative Commons Attribution (CC BY) license (https:// creativecommons.org/licenses/by/ 4.0/).

1. Introduction

Apgar scores, measured at 1 and 5 min after birth, have been used worldwide as a newborn viability and vitality evaluation tool for more than 60 years. Although the sensitivity and predictive values of this measure have been questioned in recent decades [1], it remains the only tool for a fast and easy evaluation of newborns. The Apgar score ranges from 0 to 10, and a low score is usually defined as <7 [2,3], although other cutoff values have been used in different studies [4,5]. The score given at one minute (Apgar 1) is considered an indicator of antepartum complications associated with infant mortality, morbidity, and development, especially in the short term [6,7]. The score given at five minutes (Apgar 5) has been shown to highly correlate with neonatal survival and long-term morbidity in general, and it is considered an indicator of antepartum complications and prenatal environment, regardless of gestational age at birth [5–8]. A low Apgar 5 score may be indicative of a substantial intrapartum hypoxic–ischemic event and other neonatal complications [9], and it is therefore associated with offspring neurological development; function; and morbidity, including neonatal seizures and intracranial hemorrhage, cerebral palsy [4,10,11], neurological disability, and epilepsy [12,13]. The main risk factor for these neurological complications and morbidities is prematurity [14–16]. The brain of premature newborns is not fully developed, as well as the lungs and other systems, making them more susceptible and vulnerable to harmful exposures. Due to the intensive care and interventions they undergo, the rates of many neurological complications, with possible long-term consequences, are higher among offspring born premature, and the risk increases with earlier gestational age at delivery [17–19].

The use of low Apgar 5 scores for the prediction of long-term health has been questioned [20], and studies present inconsistent findings. While Diepeveen et al. [11] found a low Apgar 5 score to be associated with language impairment at early school age, Blackman et al. [21] found no association with neurodevelopment at age 5, and Seidman et al. [22] found a poor correlation between low Apgar scores and intelligence scores at age 17. We therefore aimed to deepen the understanding of the potential predictive value of low Apgar scores and offspring neurological morbidity throughout childhood, and to study this possible association among offspring born at term and preterm.

2. Experimental Section

2.1. Study Design

A population-based retrospective cohort analysis was performed, and it included all offspring born between the years 1991 and 2021 and discharged alive from the Soroka University Medical Center (SUMC). SUMC is a single tertiary-level hospital providing care for the entire southern region of Israel, with labor and delivery units, adjacent to neonatal intensive care units, and general and pediatric emergency and critical care units. SUMC serves a population of 1.5 million residents, and with >17,000 births/year in recent years, it is among the largest birth centers in Israel.

The independent variable was defined as a low (<7) 5 min Apgar score based on maternal delivery chart. The SUMC perinatal computerized dataset consists of information recorded directly following delivery by an obstetrician. Coding is performed following the assessment of prenatal care records in addition to routine hospital documents.

The outcome variable (event) was defined as the first pediatric hospitalization of the offspring up to the age of 18 years, with any neurological diagnoses (the index hospitalization). Neurological diagnoses were predefined using a list of the International Classification of Diseases (ICD-9) codes. A list of the grouped diagnoses and ICD-9 codes is presented in Supplementary Table S1. The pediatric hospitalization dataset includes ICD-9 codes for all medical diagnoses, as well as demographic information. All diagnoses were grouped according to systems and organs, and a list of all neurological morbidities was created. The perinatal dataset was cross-linked and matched with the pediatric hospitalization dataset based on maternal and offspring personal identifying numbers. Follow-up time was calculated from birth to an event or until censored. Censoring occurred in the case of death (during hospitalization, not neurological related), reaching age 18, or at the end of the study period. Only the first hospitalization with any neurological diagnoses for each offspring was included in the analyses. For instance, in case the offspring was hospitalized for feeding intolerance or UTI, these hospitalizations were not included; however, if there was a hospitalization due to seizures, this was defined as the event, or index hospitalization, even though this may have been the second or third hospitalization for this offspring.

In order to reduce potential confounding effects, multiple gestations and newborns with major congenital malformations or chromosomal abnormalities were excluded from the study, as well as newborns with missing 5 min Apgar scores.

2.2. Statistical Analysis

Statistical analysis was performed using STATA (version 12.0, https://www.stata.com/, accessed on 27 March 2022) and SPSS (version 26.0, https://www.ibm.com/products/spss-statistics, accessed on 27 March 2022) software. Assumptions were two sided with $\alpha = 0.05$ and $\beta = 0.2$.

Initial analysis compared background, pregnancy, and perinatal characteristics between the study groups (low or normal Apgar 5 scores), using Fisher exact χ^2 test for categorical variables and t-test for comparison of means of continuous variables with normal distribution. Background, pregnancy, and perinatal characteristics included maternal age, parity, gestational age at delivery, mode of delivery, pregnancy complications, and offspring gender.

Incidence rates of neurological-related hospitalizations were calculated, and time to the first hospitalization per diagnoses group was compared between the study groups using hazard ratio (HR), which were the results of unadjusted Cox regressions. If more than one diagnosis was present per offspring during the index hospitalization, all diagnoses were included in the univariable comparison between the groups.

Kaplan–Meier survival curves were constructed, and the cumulative neurological hospitalization incidence (with any neurological morbidity) was compared between the groups using the Cox–Mantel log-rank test. The Kaplan–Meier curves were also used to assess the proportionality assumption of the risk between the study groups.

In order to identify possible confounding variables, the following were each tested for their associations with the outcome variable: background; pregnancy; and perinatal characteristics, which were statistically different between the study groups based on initial tests. In case the variable was associated with both the study group and the outcome, it was entered into the multivariable model. If, due to the inclusion of the variable, the main effect (adjusted HR) changed by >10%, the variable was included in the final model. Variables with clinical importance, such as maternal age, and offspring year of birth, which represents different changes over the study period, were also included in the multivariable analysis, even though they may have not changed the effect by >10%.

The multivariable Cox survival models were used to compare the independent risk for neurological-related morbidity based on presence of a low Apgar 5 score, and adjusted HRs were calculated. Separate multivariable models were used to study the risk specifically among term and preterm newborns (<37 gestational weeks; as well as specifically among <32 and <28 gestational weeks). The final models were selected based on the best model fit and lowest −2 log likelihood.

The study protocol was approved by the SUMC institutional review board (committee #0438-15-SOR), and informed consent was exempt.

3. Results

Between the years 1991 and 2021, there were 356,356 singleton deliveries without malformations at Soroka Medical Center, of which 6791 (2.0%) were excluded due to missing data on the 5 min Apgar score, resulting in a study population of 349,385 offspring. A low Apgar 5 score was present in 2030 (0.6%) newborns, referred to as the 'exposed group'. Among this group, the score was 0–4 in 657 newborns, and 1953 scored 5–7.

The background data of the study population are presented in Table 1. As compared to the normal Apgar 5 group, exposed newborns were more likely to be males, be delivered earlier, have a lower mean birthweight, and follow pregnancies complicated with maternal hypertensive disorders or gestational diabetes mellitus.

Table 1. Characteristics of the study population with normal or low Apgar 5 scores.

Characteristics	Low Apgar (<7)	Normal Apgar	χ^2 or t Values and Degree of Freedom (d.f), p	OR (95%CI)
	n (%)	n (%)		
	1551 (0.4)	347,051 (99.6)		
Maternal age (mean ± SD)	28.44 ± 6.2	28.25 ± 5.8	t = −1.1 (d.f = 1559), p = 0.23	
Parity			χ^2 = 56 (d.f = 2), p < 0.001	
1	485 (31.1)	84,493 (24.3)		
2–4	669 (43.2)	180,433 (52.0)		
≥5	396 (25.5)	82,078 (23.7)		
Gestational age, week (mean ± SD)	37.62 ± 3.7	39.10 ± 1.7	t = 16 (d.f = 1551), p < 0.001	
Preterm delivery (<37 weeks)	366 (23.6)	21,767 (6.3)	χ^2 = 780 (d.f = 1), p < 0.001	4.62 (4.11–5.20)
Gestational diabetes mellitus	102 (6.6)	16,681 (4.8)	χ^2 = 3 (d.f = 1), p = 0.002	1.34 (1.14–1.71)
Hypertensive disorders of pregnancy	128 (8.3)	16,177 (4.7)	χ^2 = 44 (d.f = 1)	1.84 (1.53–2.21)
Chorioamnionitis	128 (6.3)	1560 (0.4)	χ^2 = 1439 (d.f = 1), p < 0.001	14.91 (12.39–17.96)
Gender			χ^2 = 21 (d.f = 1), p < 0.001	1.27 (1.15–1.40)
Male	882 (56.9)	176,921 (51.0)		
Female	669 (43.1)	170,136 (49.0)		
Birthweight, g (mean ± SD)	2902 ± 773	3215 ± 492	t = 16 (d.f = 1555), p < 0.001	
Low birthweight (≤2500 g)	352 (22.7)	21,754 (6.3)	χ^2 = 701 (d.f = 1), p < 0.001	4.39 (3.89–4.95)
Non-reassuring fetal heart rate	406 (26.2)	18,283 (5.3)	χ^2 = 1330 (d.f = 1), p < 0.001	6.38 (5.69–7.15)
Small for gestational age	125 (8.1)	15,044 (4.3)	χ^2 = 51 (d.f = 1), p < 0.001	1.93 (1.61–2.32)
Cesarean delivery	798 (51.5)	48,458 (14.0)	χ^2 = 1788 (d.f = 1), p < 0.0001	6.53 (5.91–7.22)
Labor induction	273 (17.6)	74,220 (21.4)	χ^2 = 13 (d.f = 1), p < 0.001	0.78 (0.69–0.89)
Meconium-stained amniotic fluid	286 (18.4)	41,802 (12.0)	χ^2 = 59 (d.f =1), p < 0.001	1.65 (1.45–1.88)

The study population was followed for an average of 10.8 ± 6.5 years and 7.8 ± 6.4 years (normal and low 5 min Apgar groups, respectively, p < 0.001). The Kaplan–Meier analysis (shown in Figure 1) presents the significant difference in survival between the study groups (log-rank, p < 0.001), indicating that the offspring with a low 5 min Apgar score tended to have shorter survival. The survival curves present the proportionality of survival between the two study groups.

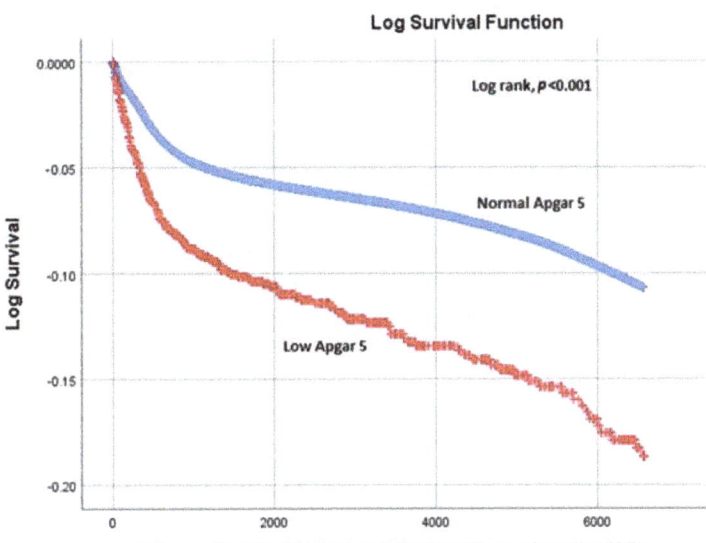

Figure 1. Cumulative survival by study group.

During the follow-up period, 175 (11.3%) offspring with low Apgar 5 scores were hospitalized with neurological-related morbidities as compared to 25,898 (7.5%) in the normal Apgar score group (hazard ratio, HR = 1.84; 95% confidence interval, CI 1.58–2.13). Selected neurological morbidities with normal or low 5 min Apgar scores are presented in Table 2. Offspring with a low Apgar score were more likely to be hospitalized with any of the neurological morbidities, including epilepsy and movement disorders, cerebral palsy, and developmental disorders.

Table 2. Selected neurological morbidities with normal or low 5 min Apgar scores.

	Low Apgar (<7)	Normal Apgar	Unadjusted Hazard Ratio; 95%CI
	n (%) 1551 (0.4)	n (%) 347,051 (99.6)	
Autism	3 (0.2)	228 (0.1)	3.77; 1.21–11.77
Epilepsy and movement disorders	83 (5.4)	10,470 (3.0)	2.07; 1.67–2.57
Cerebral palsy	27 (1.7)	664 (0.2)	11.07; 7.53–16.27
Developmental disorders	30 (1.9)	3056 (0.9)	1.91; 1.52–2.41
Degenerative disorders	19 (1.2)	688 (0.2)	7.07; 4.48–11.15
Psychiatric and emotional disorders	72 (4.6)	9983 (2.9)	2.38; 1.66–3.41
Total neurological-related hospitalizations	175 (11.3)	25,898 (7.5)	1.84; 1.58–2.13

Among offspring born at term (n = 299,614), the rates of neurological-related hospitalizations were 125 (10.6%) vs. 23,550 (7.2%) among low and normal Apgar 5 scores, respectively (OR = 1.51; 95%CI 1.26–1.82). Among preterm-born offspring (<37 gestational weeks, n = 22,133), the rates of hospitalizations were 50 (13.7%) vs. 2341 (10.8%) among low and normal Apgar 5 scores, respectively (OR = 1.31; 95%CI 0.97–1.78). The power to test the studied association among preterm <37 gestational weeks was 43%.

In the multivariable survival models presented in Table 3, for the entire study population, offspring born with a low 5 min Apgar score were 1.61 times more likely to be hospitalized with neurological morbidities after adjusting for preterm births, maternal age, delivery mode, chorioamnionitis, and maternal hypertension or diabetes (adjusted hazard ratio (Adj. HR) = 1.61; 95%CI 1.39–1.87). This association was present specifically among term-born offspring (Adj. HR = 1.70; 95%CI 1.43–2.03) but not among preterm-born offspring (<37 gestational weeks) (adj. HR = 1.18; 95%CI 0.88–1.57).

Table 3. Total neurological-related hospitalizations and low vs. normal Apgar scores *.

	Adjusted Hazard Ratios *		
	All	Preterm	Term
Low Vs. Normal Apgar 5	1.61; 1.39–1.87	1.16; 0.87–1.54	1.70; 1.42–2.02
Hypertensive disorders	1.10; 1.04–1.15	1.11; 0.99–1.25	1.09; 1.07–1.15
Gestational diabetes mellitus	1.03; 0.97–1.09	0.95; 0.78–1.15	1.04; 0.98–1.11
Cesarean vs. vaginal delivery	1.10; 1.06–1.14	1.02; 0.94–1.12	1.11; 1.07–1.16
Chorioamnionitis	1.11; 0.96–1.28	1.11; 0.90–1.36	1.09; 0.89–1.35
Preterm delivery **	1.44; 1.38–1.50	-	-

* All models additionally adjusted for maternal age and year of birth. ** Among the preterm and term models, gestational age adjusted for instead of preterm delivery.

A stratified analysis among offspring born preterm is presented in Table 4. The stratified analysis reveals that the lack of association between a low Apgar score and neurological-related hospitalization among offspring born preterm is due to the earlier gestational ages; among offspring born <32 gestational age, a low Apgar score was not associated with neurological-related morbidities, either in the univariable analysis or after adjusting for maternal age. Specifically, among offspring born <28 gestational age, although not statistically significant, a low Apgar score was associated with a lower risk of hospitalization.

Table 4. Incidence and multivariable analysis for total neurological-related hospitalizations among offspring born preterm *.

Gestational Age at Delivery	Apgar	n	Neurological-Related Hospitalization	OR; 95%CI	Adjusted HR; 95%CI *
<28	Low Apgar (<7)	381	7 (1.8)	0.10; 0.05–0.21	0.59; 0.27–1.28
	Normal Apgar	604	97 (16.1)		
28–32	Low Apgar (<7)	124	11 (11.8)	0.92; 0.53–1.59	1.35; 0.80–2.29
	Normal Apgar	2148	274 (12.8)		
32–36	Low Apgar (<7)	421	51 (12.1)	1.36; 1.01–1.82	1.72; 1.30–2.27
	Normal Apgar	45,712	4216 (9.2)		

* Adjusted for maternal age.

4. Discussion

In this large population-based cohort with a long follow-up period, a low 5 min Apgar score was independently associated with pediatric neurological hospitalizations. This association was not present among preterm-born offspring. Although the possibility of insufficient power cannot be ruled out in the latter cases, it is also possible that other factors, such as those possibly leading to early delivery, the intensive interventions following delivery, and the prematurity itself, are the ones increasing the risk for neurological morbidities, regardless of the Apgar score.

Apgar scores have long been established as a prediction tool for short-term neonatal survival and morbidity. Their value in the prediction of long-term outcome has been questioned in recent years.

Low Apgar scores have been associated with perinatal asphyxia and immaturity or impairment of the central nervous system [23]. These postpartum complications may be involved in neurological morbidity mechanisms, from cerebral palsy (CP) to developmental and language impairments [11,23]. Prematurity is known to be associated with an increased risk for long-term morbidities [24] due to both the immaturity of different systems, specifically the lungs and the brain, and the possible side effects of the intensive care and iatrogenic interventions often critical for life support. As opposed to those of term newborns, preterm newborns' Apgar scores may represent developmental achievements rather than fetal compromise [25]. It is possible that it is for this reason that a low Apgar score among preterm-born offspring was not independently associated with long-term complications. It is also possible that the current cohort includes relatively healthy, resilient offspring, who, although were born with a low Apgar score, were discharged alive from the hospital. This too may explain the lack of association and possibly suggest a protective association between low Apgar scores and neurological-related hospitalizations among preterm- and, specifically, extreme preterm-born offspring.

Other studies have also reached similar conclusions; Jensen et al. [9] found a low 5 min Apgar score to be associated with CP or death across all gestational ages; however, the association was weaker with deceasing gestational age at birth. Low Apgar scores have been found to be associated with an increased risk for infantile seizures, specifically among full-term and normal-birth-weight infants [26], and Lie et al. [23] found a stronger association between low Apgar scores and CP among normal- as compared to low-birth-weight offspring.

Since this study was of a retrospective nature, several limitations were present. The first limitation is related to the subjective nature of the Apgar score being assigned by the staff, such as a midwife or a pediatrician. Data regarding the medical staff assigning the Apgar score were unavailable for analysis. Inter-observer Apgar scoring variability is expected [27], and there is a possibility that different medical staff members tend to grade higher or lower than others. However, there is no reason to suspect that this distribution was associated with the risk for neurological morbidity likelihood later in life. Other factors that are known to be associated with Apgar scores, such as congenital malformations, gestational age, and mode of delivery, have been either excluded or accounted for in the multivariable analysis.

This study's aim was to evaluate the predictive value of a low 5 min Apgar score in relation to pediatric neurological morbidities. However, since cases of neonatal deaths were excluded from the long-term follow-up and only newborns that were discharged alive from the hospital following delivery were included, a survival bias is present in our findings, since newborns with the lowest Apgar scores are underrepresented in the cohort. Since the cohort includes relatively 'healthy' offspring, our results are probably an under-estimation of the true association between low Apgar scores and neurological morbidities.

This study has several strengths, including the long follow-up period, which enabled the associations between low Apgar scores and long-term neurological-related pediatric hospitalizations to be addressed. Moreover, due to the large cohort size, we were able to study less-frequent neurological morbidities, as well as the association among preterm offspring, extreme preterm offspring, and twins.

According to the ACOG's 2015 statement [23], low Apgar 5 score monitoring may identify needs for focused educational programs and improvement in systems of perinatal care.

5. Conclusions

Although Apgar scores are not intended for the prediction of neurological morbidities, our findings suggest Apgar scores may be used, possibly independently or in combination with other measures, as a predictor of later neurological morbidities among term-born but not preterm-born offspring. The early detection of newborns at risk for long-term adverse health outcomes can lead to early treatment and reduce the odds of long-term adverse health effects.

Supplementary Materials: The following supporting information can be downloaded at: https://www.mdpi.com/article/10.3390/jcm11071922/s1; Table S1: Neurological diagnoses and ICD-9 codes.

Author Contributions: Conceptualization, T.W. and E.S.; methodology, T.W. and E.S.; software, T.W.; formal analysis, T.W.; writing—original draft preparation, T.W.; writing—review and editing, E.S. All authors have read and agreed to the published version of the manuscript.

Funding: This research received no external funding.

Institutional Review Board Statement: The study was conducted in accordance with the Declaration of Helsinki, and approved by the Institutional Review Board of Soroka University Medical Center (protocol #0357-19-SOR, October 2019).

Informed Consent Statement: Patient consent was waived since the analysis was based on a de-identified computerized database.

Data Availability Statement: Data will be made available by request and according to IRB restrictions.

Conflicts of Interest: The authors declare no conflict of interest.

References

1. ACOG Committee on Obstetric Practice. American Academy of Pediatrics Committee on Fetus and Newborn. Use and Abuse of the Apgar Score. In *Compendium of Selected Publications*; No. 174; American College of Obstetricians and Gynecologists: Washington, DC, USA, 1996.
2. Salustiano, E.M.; Campos, J.A.; Ibidi, S.M.; Ruano, R.; Zugaib, M. Low Apgar scores at 5 minutes in a low risk population: Maternal and obstetrical factors and postnatal outcome. *Rev. Assoc. Med. Bras.* **2012**, *58*, 587–593. [CrossRef]
3. Svenvik, M.; Brudin, L.; Blomberg, M. Preterm Birth: A Prominent Risk Factor for Low Apgar Scores. *BioMed Res. Int.* **2015**, *2015*, 978079. [CrossRef] [PubMed]
4. Li, J.; Cnattingius, S.; Gissler, M.; Vestergaard, M.; Obel, C.; Ahrensberg, J.; Olsen, J. The 5-minute Apgar score as a predictor of childhood cancer: A population-based cohort study in five million children. *BMJ Open.* **2012**, *2*, 4. [CrossRef] [PubMed]
5. Phalen, A.G.; Kirkby, S.; Dysart, K. The 5-minute Apgar score: Survival and short-term outcomes in extremely low-birth-weight infants. *J. Perinat. Neonatal. Nurs.* **2012**, *26*, 166–171. [CrossRef] [PubMed]
6. Moster, D.; Lie, R.T.; Irgens, L.M.; Bjerkedal, T.; Markestad, T. The association of Apgar score with subsequent death and cerebral palsy: A population-based study in term infants. *J. Pediatr.* **2010**, *138*, 798–803. [CrossRef] [PubMed]
7. Iliodromiti, S.; Mackay, D.F.; Smith, G.C.S.; Pell, J.P.; Nelson, S.M. Apgar score and the risk of cause-specific infant mortality: A population-based cohort study. *Lancet* **2014**, *384*, 1749–1755. [CrossRef]
8. Li, F.; Wu, T.; Lei, X.; Zhang, H.; Mao, M.; Zhang, J. The Apgar score and infant mortality. *PLoS ONE* **2013**, *8*, e69072. [CrossRef]
9. Jensen, L.V.; Mathiasen, R.; Mølholm, B.; Greisen, G. Low 5-min Apgar score in moderately preterm infants; association with subsequent death and cerebral palsy: A register based Danish national study. *Acta Paediatr.* **2012**, *101*, e80–e82. [CrossRef]
10. Ehrenstein, V.; Pedersen, L.; Grijota, M.; Nielsen, G.L.; Rothman, K.J.; Sørensen, H.T. Association of Apgar score at five minutes with long-term neurologic disability and cognitive function in a prevalence study of Danish conscripts. *BMC Preg. Child.* **2009**, *9*, 14. [CrossRef] [PubMed]
11. Diepeveen, F.B.; De Kroon, M.L.; Dusseldorp, E.; Snik, A.F. Among perinatal factors, only the Apgar score is associated with specific language impairment. *Dev. Med. Child Neurol.* **2013**, *55*, 631–635. [CrossRef]
12. Ehrenstein, V. Association of Apgar scores with death and neurologic disability. *Clin. Epidemiol.* **2009**, *9*, 45–53. [CrossRef] [PubMed]
13. Sun, Y.; Vestergaard, M.; Pedersen, C.B.; Christensen, J.; Olsen, J. Apgar scores and long-term risk of epilepsy. *Epidemiology* **2006**, *17*, 296–301. [CrossRef] [PubMed]
14. Melamed, N.; Klinger, G.; Tenenbaum-Gavish, K.; Herscovici, T.; Linder, N.; Hod, M.; Yariv, Y. Short-term neonatal outcome in low-risk, spontaneous, singleton, late preterm deliveries. *Obstet. Gynecol.* **2009**, *114*, 253–260. [CrossRef] [PubMed]
15. WHO. Fact Sheets on Preterm Birth. Available online: http://www.who.int/topics/preterm_birth/en/ (accessed on 27 March 2022).
16. Hadar, O.; Sheiner, E.; Wainstock, T. The Association between Delivery of Small-for-Gestational-Age Neonate and Their Risk for Long-Term Neurological Morbidity. *J. Clin. Med.* **2020**, *9*, 3199. [CrossRef]
17. Crump, C. An overview of adult health outcomes after preterm birth. *Early Hum. Dev.* **2020**, *150*, 105187. [CrossRef] [PubMed]
18. Luu, T.M.; Rehman Mian, M.O.; Nuyt, A.M. Long-Term Impact of Preterm Birth: Neurodevelopmental and Physical Health Outcomes. *Clin. Perinatol.* **2017**, *44*, 305–314. [CrossRef] [PubMed]
19. Zer, S.; Wainstock, T.; Sheiner, E.; Miodownik, S.; Pariente, G. Identifying the Critical Threshold for Long-Term Pediatric Neurological Hospitalizations of the Offspring in Preterm Delivery. *J. Clin. Med.* **2021**, *10*, 2919. [CrossRef]
20. Ruth, V.J.; Raivio, K.O. Perinatal brain damage: Predictive value of metabolic acidosis and the Apgar score. *BMJ* **1988**, *297*, 24–27. [CrossRef]
21. Blackman, J.A. The value of Apgar scores in predicting developmental outcome at age five. *J. Perinatol.* **1988**, *8*, 206–210.
22. Seidman, D.S.; Paz, I.; Laor, A.; Gale, R.; Stevenson, D.K.; Danon, Y.L. Apgar scores and cognitive performance at 17 years of age. *Obstet. Gynecol.* **1991**, *77*, 875–878.
23. Lie, K.K.; Grøholt, E.K.; Eskild, A. Association of cerebral palsy with Apgar score in low and normal birthweight infants: Population based cohort study. *BMJ* **2010**, *341*, c4990. [CrossRef] [PubMed]
24. Newman, D.E.; Paamoni-Keren, O.; Press, F.; Wiznitzer, A.; Mazor, M.; Sheiner, E. Neonatal outcome in preterm deliveries between 23 and 27 weeks' gestation with and without preterm premature rupture of membranes. *Arch. Gynecol. Obstet.* **2009**, *280*, 7–11. [CrossRef] [PubMed]
25. Catlin, E.A.; Carpenter, M.W.; Brann, B.S.; Mayfield, S.R.; Shaul, P.W.; Goldstein, M.; Oh, W. The Apgar score revisited: Influence of gestational age. *J. Pediatr.* **1986**, *109*, 865–868. [CrossRef]

26. Eun, S.; Lee, J.M.; Yi, D.Y.; Lee, N.M.; Kim, H.; Yun, S.W.; Lim, I.; Choi, E.S.; Chae, S.A. Assessment of the association between Apgar scores and seizures in infants less than 1 year old. *Seizure* **2016**, *37*, 48–54. [CrossRef] [PubMed]
27. Committee on Obstetric Practice American Academy of Pediatrics-Committee on Fetus and Newborn. Committee Opinion No. 644: The Apgar Score. *Obstet Gynecol.* **2015**, *4*, e52–e55. [CrossRef]

Article

Prematurity and Long-Term Respiratory Morbidity—What Is the Critical Gestational Age Threshold?

Gil Gutvirtz [1,*], Tamar Wainstock [2], Eyal Sheiner [1] and Gali Pariente [1]

[1] Department of Obstetrics and Gynecology, Soroka University Medical Center, Ben-Gurion University of the Negev, Beer-Sheva 8457108, Israel; sheiner@bgu.ac.il (E.S.); galipa@bgu.ac.il (G.P.)
[2] Department of Public Health, Faculty of Health Sciences, Ben-Gurion University of the Negev, Beer-Sheva 8457108, Israel; wainstoc@bgu.ac.il
* Correspondence: giltzik@gmail.com

Abstract: Respiratory morbidity is a hallmark complication of prematurity. Children born preterm are exposed to both short- and long-term respiratory morbidity. This study aimed to investigate whether a critical gestational age threshold exists for significant long-term respiratory morbidity. A 23-year, population-based cohort analysis was performed comparing singleton deliveries at a single tertiary medical center. A comparison of four gestational age groups was performed according to the WHO classification: term ($\geq$37.0 weeks, reference group), moderate to late preterm (32.0–36.6 weeks), very preterm (28.0–31.6 weeks) and extremely preterm (24.0–27.6 weeks). Hospitalizations of the offspring up to the age of 18 years involving respiratory morbidities were evaluated. A Kaplan–Meier survival curve was used to compare cumulative hospitalization incidence between the groups. A Cox proportional hazards model was used to control for confounders and time to event. Overall, 220,563 singleton deliveries were included: 93.6% term deliveries, 6% moderate to late preterm, 0.4% very preterm and 0.1% extremely preterm. Hospitalizations involving respiratory morbidity were significantly higher in children born preterm (12.7% in extremely preterm children, 11.7% in very preterm, 7.0% in late preterm vs. 4.7% in term, $p < 0.001$). The Kaplan–Meier survival curve demonstrated a significantly higher cumulative incidence of respiratory-related hospitalizations in the preterm groups (log-rank, $p < 0.001$). In the Cox regression model, delivery before 32 weeks had twice the risk of long-term respiratory morbidity. Searching for a specific gestational age threshold, the slope for hospitalization rate was attenuated beyond 30 weeks' gestation. In our population, it seems that 30 weeks' gestation may be the critical threshold for long-term respiratory morbidity of the offspring, as the risk for long-term respiratory-related hospitalization seems to be attenuated beyond this point until term.

Keywords: prematurity; gestational age; threshold; respiratory morbidity; pediatric hospitalization

1. Introduction

Prematurity is defined by the WHO as a birth before 37 completed weeks' gestation and is associated with significant infant mortality and morbidity [1,2]. Worldwide, the preterm birth rate is estimated to be approximately 11% [3,4]. The WHO defines three subcategories for prematurity according to gestational age (GA) at birth: extremely preterm (less than 28 weeks' gestation), very preterm (28–32 weeks' gestation) and moderate to late preterm (32–36 weeks' gestation). This classification mainly reflects the offspring prognosis, as mortality rates correlate with GA [5]. Infants born at or before 28 weeks of gestation have the highest mortality with reported death rates of approximately 50 percent [6], although infant survival rates have improved over the years, especially in high-income countries [7]. Nevertheless, even among tertiary neonatal centers in the United States, there is a variation in mortality that ranges between 5% to 36% for all GAs and 13–73% for infants less than 25 weeks' gestation [8]. One of the main causes of early infant death is respiratory disorders [9,10] especially in extremely preterm infants. Preterm birth interferes with the development of the lung and may render it less effective as a gas exchanger or may make it more susceptible to disease by changing the "program" that determines its development [11]. Those who survive may suffer short-term complications (e.g., respiratory distress syndrome (RDS), patent ductus arteriosus (PDA) and bronchopulmonary dysplasia (BPD)) during the neonatal period [12] and long-term sequelae including repeated hospitalizations [13,14], chronic respiratory diseases [15–17] and neurodevelopmental disabilities such as cerebral palsy (CP) [18,19].

Respiratory morbidity is one of the most prominent complications of prematurity, starting with RDS with increasing incidence as GA decreases [12] and followed by BPD as a later respiratory complication. While these complications are short-term in appearance, they are known to have long-term consequences on lung function [20], and the outcome of poor lung development depends on the type and severity of the insult as well as the lung developmental stage at which it occurs [21].

As respiratory morbidity is one of the devastating outcomes of prematurity, we opted to investigate the correlation between the degree of prematurity and long-term respiratory morbidity of the offspring in order to establish a critical cut-off at which the long-term respiratory morbidity of the offspring would be higher.

2. Methods

This was a population-based, retrospective study conducted at the Soroka University Medical Center (SUMC) between the years 1991 and 2014. It included all singleton deliveries occurring within this time period at SUMC and followed offspring hospitalizations in SUMC until 18 years of age.

The institutional review board (SUMC IRB Committee) approved the study that has been performed, which is in accordance with the ethical standards laid down by the 1964 Declaration of Helsinki and its later amendments (Helsinki Declaration 1975, revision 2013).

The SUMC is the largest birth center in the country and the sole tertiary hospital in the Negev area that includes a neonatal intensive care unit (NICU) and pediatric wards.

The area has experienced positive immigration over the last two decades, with increasing annual birth rates reaching approximately 15,000 by the end of the study period. As the only hospital in the area, children born in the SUMC are also expected to be hospitalized in the hospital's pediatric wards, if indicated.

A comparison of 4 gestational age groups was performed according to the WHO classification [1]: term births ($\geq$37.0 weeks), moderate to late preterm (32.0–36.6 weeks), very preterm (28.0–31.6 weeks) and extremely preterm (24.0–27.6 weeks).

We excluded cases of multiple pregnancies and congenital malformations, as both factors are associated with preterm delivery and chronic health problems. Perinatal mortality cases were also excluded from the long-term analysis.

Maternal characteristics included maternal age and background morbidity (pre-gestational diabetes and chronic hypertension). Selective pregnancy complications were also recorded including gestational diabetes mellitus (GDM) and hypertensive disorders (preeclampsia with and without severe features and eclampsia).

The primary outcome variables included respiratory-related hospitalizations of the offspring up to the age of 18 years, as recorded in hospital records, using predefined diagnoses of ICD-9 codes detailed in the Table S1. Secondary outcomes assessed included adverse perinatal outcomes such as intra-amniotic infection rates (a clinical diagnosis made by an obstetrician during labor defined by a combination of common clinical criteria for chorioamnionitis, including maternal fever, maternal and fetal tachycardia, uterine tenderness and foul amniotic fluid), low Apgar scores (<7) given to the neonate at 5 min, small for gestational age (SGA), defined as birthweight <5th percentile for gestational age and gender, and cesarean delivery rates.

Follow-up time was defined as time to event (respiratory-related hospitalization, as first diagnosis or background diagnosis) and ended at either first hospitalization, child death (during hospitalization for unrelated morbidity), reaching age of 18 or at the end of the study period, whichever milestone was reached first.

We used 2 distinct hospital databases in order to merge and cross-link maternal and offspring data The first is the computerized obstetrics and gynecology department database, which consists of maternal and obstetrical information recorded at the mothers' admission to the delivery room after assessing medical prenatal care records and immediately following delivery by an obstetrician. The second is the pediatric hospitalization database, which includes demographic information and ICD-9 codes for all medical diagnoses made during hospitalization in any of the pediatric departments at the SUMC. In the SUMC, all records are routinely reviewed by experienced medical secretaries for accuracy and completeness prior to entering them into the databases.

Statistical Analysis

We used the SPSS package 23rd edition (IBM/SPSS, Chicago, IL, USA) to perform the study's statistical analysis. Background, clinical and outcome variables were compared between the study groups using χ^2 tests for categorical variables and Student's t test for continuous variables with normal distribution. Kaplan–Meier survival curves were used to compare cumulative respiratory-related hospitalization incidences during follow-up time according to gestational age at birth, divided into the four subgroups characterized above, and differences between curves were assessed using log-rank test. A Cox regression model was used to investigate the association between gestational age at birth and pediatric respiratory-related hospitalization risk. The model was adjusted based on the univariate analysis and clinically relevant variables including follow-up time, maternal age, mode of delivery, birthweight, diabetes mellitus, hypertensive disorders and presence of intra-amniotic infection (clinically diagnosed chorioamnionitis). Term deliveries were used as the reference group for the comparison. All analyses were two-sided. A p-value < 0.05 was considered statistically significant.

3. Results

During the study period, 220,563 singleton deliveries met the inclusion criteria. Of those, 93.6% (n = 206,361) were born at term, 6% (n = 13,308) were moderate to late preterm, 0.4% (n = 776) were very preterm and 0.1% (n = 118) were extremely preterm

Maternal characteristics and immediate perinatal outcomes according to the different gestational age groups are presented in Table 1. A statistically significant difference in maternal age was noted between groups; however, it was clinically irrelevant. Incidence of hypertensive disorders was highest in women who delivered very preterm and lowest in women who delivered at term. Incidence of intra-amniotic infection and cesarean deliveries decreased progressively as gestational age increased. Diabetes was more common in women from the preterm groups except for those who delivered extremely preterm.

Table 2 summarizes the selected respiratory morbidities and total hospitalization rate for the four study groups according to prematurity severity. Offspring born preterm had a significantly higher respiratory-related hospitalization rate compared to term offspring, as the hospitalization rate increased with decreasing gestational age (4.7%, 7.0%, 11.7% and 12.7% for offspring born in term delivery, moderate to late PTB, very PTB and extremely PTB, respectively, p < 0.001 for trends).

Table 1. Maternal characteristics and pregnancy outcomes according to gestational age.

Maternal Characteristics	Extremely Preterm (24.0–27.6) N = 118	Very Preterm (28.0–31.6) N = 776	Moderate to Late Preterm (32.0–36.6) N = 13,308	Term Delivery (≥37.0) N = 206,361	p Value [a]
Maternal age (mean ± SD, years)	28.4 ± 6.3	28.3 ± 6.3	28.3 ± 6.2	28.2 ± 5.7	<0.001
Diabetes mellitus [b] (%)	0.0	6.2	8.2	5.3	<0.001
Hypertensive disorders [c] (%)	8.5	19.1	12.9	4.7	<0.001
Induction of labor (%)	10.2	9.3	23.1	27.6	<0.001
Intra-amniotic infection (%)	33.1	14.3	2.6	0.3	<0.001
Cesarean Delivery (%)	51.7	52.8	31.0	12.7	<0.001
Low Apgar at 5 min (<7) (%)	14.4	6.2	2.5	1.4	<0.001
Gestational age at delivery (mean ± SD, weeks)	26.4 ± 0.7	30.0 ± 1.0	35.2 ± 1.1	39.4 ± 1.2	<0.001
Birthweight (mean ± SD, grams)	1096 ± 601	1644 ± 633	2540 ± 495	3270 ± 445	<0.001
SGA [d] (%)	3.4	1.8	3.6	4.4	<0.001

[a] Calculated for all groups using the chi square test for trends; [b] including pre-gestational and gestational diabetes; [c] including chronic hypertension, gestational hypertension, preeclampsia with or without severe features and eclampsia; [d] SGA = small for gestational age, defined as birthweight <5th percentile for gestational age and gender.

Table 2. Selected long-term respiratory morbidities in children (up to the age of 18 years) according to gestational age at birth.

Respiratory Morbidity	Extremely Preterm (24.0–27.6) N = 118	Very Preterm (28.0–31.6) N = 776	Moderate to Late Preterm (32.0–36.6) N = 13,308	Term Delivery (≥37.0) N = 206,361	p Value [a]
Asthma (%)	3.4	5.2	3.4	2.5	<0.001
Pleural disease (%)	0.0	0.4	0.1	0.1	0.022
Obstructive sleep apnea (OSA) (%)	1.7	1.3	0.9	0.7	0.002
Other * (%)	8.5	6.6	3.0	1.9	<0.001
Total respiratory hospitalizations (%)	12.7	11.7	7.0	4.7	<0.001

[a] Calculated for all groups using the chi square test for trends. * Detailed in the supplementary table.

Mean age at hospitalization for offspring born at 24–28 weeks' gestational age was 10.2 +/− 6.6 years. A total of 12.7% of the cases occurred by the age of 1 year, and 30.5% by the age of 5 years. The median age was 12.1 years. For offspring born at 28–32 weeks' gestational age, the mean age at hospitalization was 9.13 +/− 6.4 years. A total of 11.9% of the cases occurred by the age of 1 year, and 37% by the age of 5. Median age was 8.65 years. For offspring born at 32–36 weeks' gestational age, the mean age at hospitalization was 9.92 +/− 6.1 years. A total of 7.5% of the cases occurred by the age of 1 year, and 28.1% by the age of 5. The median age was 10.2 years.

The mean age at hospitalization for offspring born at term was 10.02 +/− 6.1 years. A total of 6.8% of the cases occurred by the age of 1 year, and 27.5% by the age of 5. The median age was 10.2 years.

A significant difference was noted in the age of hospitalization between age groups 28–32 and 32–36 ($p < 0.001$) and between 28–32 and term ($p < 0.001$).

Presented in Figure 1 are the Kaplan–Meier survival curves showing a progressively higher cumulative incidence of offspring respiratory-related hospitalizations as gestational age decreases. Similar survival curves of offspring born extremely and very preterm were noted, with the highest cumulative hospitalization incidence. For all gestational age groups, the sharpest incline of hospitalizations was seen by the age of 5.

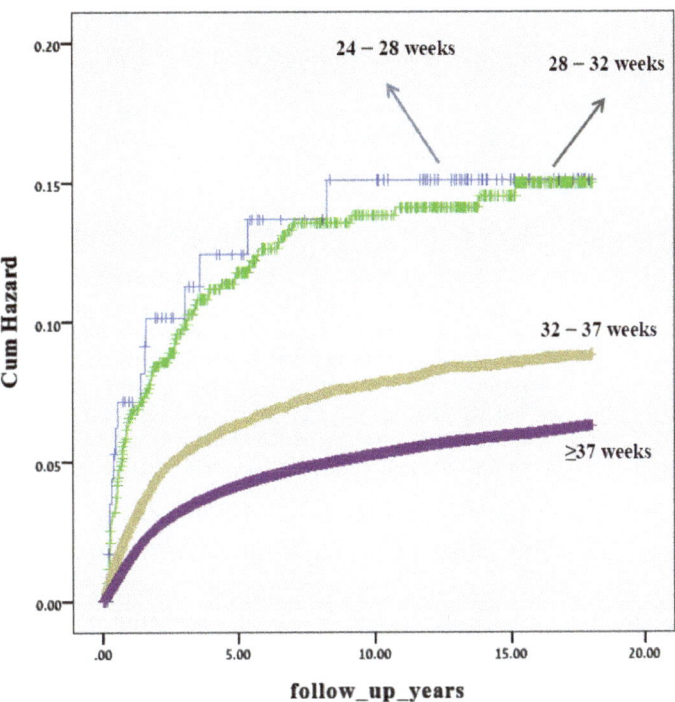

Figure 1. A Kaplan–Meier survival curve demonstrating the cumulative incidence of respiratory-related hospitalizations among study groups of different gestational age at birth.

A univariate analysis of respiratory-related hospitalization rates according to week of gestation at birth is presented in Figure 2. A general inverse relationship can be seen between gestational week at birth and incidence of respiratory-related hospitalization. At 30 weeks' gestation, the hospitalization rate drops significantly to approximately 10% (as opposed to 17% at 26 weeks); then, it is attenuated until 34 weeks, with a further decrease in hospitalization rate at 36 weeks. The curve continues to drop to its lowest point at 40 weeks (full term), although the decline is less prominent.

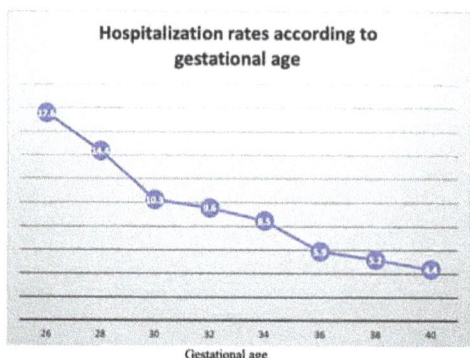

Figure 2. Respiratory-related hospitalization rates according to gestational age.

A Cox proportional hazards model is presented in Table 3. The model was constructed to adjust for follow-up time, and control for statistically significant and clinically relevant variables is described in the methods section. Using this model, prematurity (birth before 37 completed weeks) was found to be independently associated with long-term respiratory morbidity. Compared to term delivery, birth before 32 weeks' gestation (whether extremely or very preterm) carries a 2.0-fold risk for long-term respiratory morbidity, while birth at moderate to late preterm (32.0–36.6 weeks) carries a 1.3-fold risk for long-term respiratory morbidity. The critical threshold beyond which long-term respiratory morbidity decreased is 30 days.

Table 3. Multivariable analysis of long-term risk for respiratory-related hospitalizations according to gestational age.

Gestational Age	Adjusted Hazard Ratio (aHR) *	Confidence Interval (95%)	p Value
Term delivery (reference) (37–42 weeks)	1	-	-
Moderate to late preterm (32–37 weeks)	1.29	1.20–1.39	<0.01
Very preterm (28–32 weeks)	2.02	1.62–2.52	<0.01
Extremely preterm (24–28 weeks)	2.04	1.21–3.44	<0.01

* Adjusted for maternal age, birthweight, diabetes mellitus, hypertensive disorders, presence of intra-amniotic infection and mode of delivery.

Repeated hospitalizations of the offspring were also evaluated. We found the mean re-hospitalization rate decreased with increasing gestational age, from 20% in extremely premature infants (24–28 weeks' gestation) to 16% in the very preterm group (28–32 weeks), 10% in the moderate to late preterm group (32–37 weeks) and finally decreasing to only 6% in term infants (≥37 weeks).

Finally, we conducted a sub-analysis of the original cohort, dividing it to two distinct time periods—offspring born before the year 2000 (1991–1999) and those born after (2000–2014). In offspring born before the year 2000, with the exception from 26 to 28 weeks, an inverse relationship can be seen between gestational week at birth and incidence of respiratory-related hospitalization (Figure 3). At 30 weeks' gestation, the hospitalization rate is more than halved to 5.5% from 12.5% at 28 weeks. From 30 weeks' gestation, the hospitalization rate slowly declines to its lowest rate at full term (40 weeks).

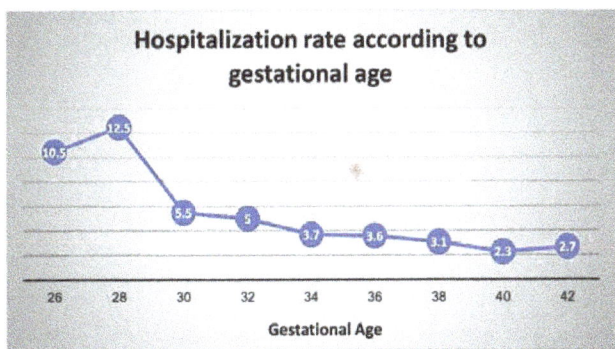

Figure 3. Respiratory-related hospitalization rates according to gestational age (offspring born before the year 2000).

A Cox regression model for this cohort, adjusted for maternal age, mode of delivery, birthweight, diabetes mellitus, hypertensive disorders and presence of intra-amniotic infection (clinically diagnosed chorioamnionitis), found prematurity (birth before 37 completed weeks) was independently associated with long-term respiratory morbidity. Compared to term delivery, being born extremely preterm, very preterm and moderate to late preterm carries a significant higher risk for long-term respiratory morbidity (aHR of 3.33, 2.61 and 1.32, respectively, Table 4).

Table 4. Multivariable analysis of long-term risk for respiratory-related hospitalizations according to gestational age (offspring born before the year 2000).

Gestational Age	Adjusted Hazard Ratio (aHR) *	Confidence Interval (95%)	*p* Value
Term delivery (reference) (37–42 weeks)	1	-	-
Moderate to late preterm (32–37 weeks)	1.32	1.12–1.56	<0.01
Very preterm (28–32 weeks)	2.61	1.70–4.02	<0.01
Extremely preterm (24–28 weeks)	3.33	1.50–7.39	<0.01

* Adjusted for maternal age, birthweight, diabetes mellitus, hypertensive disorders, presence of intra-amniotic infection and mode of delivery.

In offspring born after the year 2000, a general inverse relationship can once again be seen between gestational week at birth and incidence of respiratory-related hospitalization (Figure 4). The gradual decline in the hospitalization rate is attenuated from 30 weeks' gestation until 34 weeks, with a further decrease in the hospitalization rate at 36 weeks. The curve continues to drop to its lowest point at full term (40 weeks).

A similar Cox regression model for this sub-analysis, adjusted for maternal age, mode of delivery, birthweight, diabetes mellitus, hypertensive disorders and presence of intra-amniotic infection (clinically diagnosed chorioamnionitis), also found prematurity (birth before 37 completed weeks) was independently associated with long-term respiratory morbidity. Compared to term delivery, being born extremely preterm, very preterm and moderate to late preterm carries a significant higher risk for long-term respiratory morbidity (aHR of 2.04, 1.97 and 1.32, respectively, Table 5).

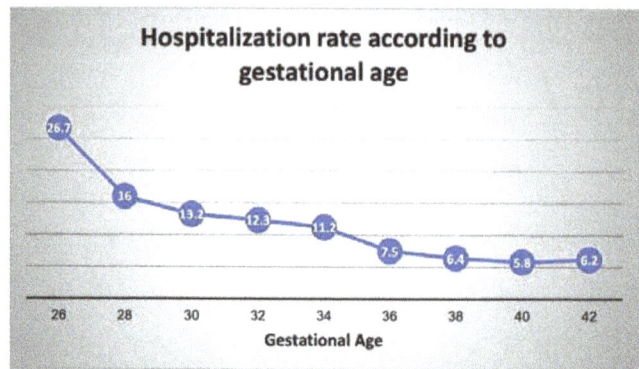

Figure 4. Respiratory-related hospitalization rates according to gestational age (offspring born after the year 2000).

Table 5. Multivariable analysis of long-term risk for respiratory-related hospitalizations according to gestational age (offspring born after the year 2000).

Gestational Age	Adjusted Hazard Ratio (aHR) *	Confidence Interval (95%)	p Value
Term delivery (reference) (37–42 weeks)	1	-	-
Moderate to late preterm (32–37 weeks)	1.32	1.21–1.44	<0.01
Very preterm (28–32 weeks)	1.97	1.52–2.55	<0.01
Extremely preterm (24–28 weeks)	2.04	1.01–4.12	0.04

* Adjusted for maternal age, birthweight, diabetes mellitus, hypertensive disorders, presence of intra-amniotic infection and mode of delivery.

4. Discussion

This large retrospective cohort study examined the long-term incidence of respiratory-related hospitalizations of children born preterm, stratified by the severity of prematurity and compared to offspring born at term. We found the risk for long-term respiratory morbidity to be increased as gestational age at birth decreased, which is in accordance with earlier literature [22–24]. Nevertheless, while most studies associate more extremely prematurity with higher rates of respiratory morbidity, they could not point out the gestational age threshold that carries the highest risk, after which the prognosis improves. Using a sub-analysis of hospitalization rates according to gestational age at birth, we found the sharpest decline at 30 weeks, which then attenuates until reaching near-term (36 weeks), where it once again declines to reach its lowest point at full term (40 weeks). 30 weeks' gestation seems to be the threshold where the risk for long-term respiratory morbidity is significantly reduced and from which point the hospitalization rate decreases to less than 10%.

This threshold is similar to that found by Copper et al. for preterm infants' survival rates. Their study, conducted in the U.S., reported that by 30 weeks of gestation, survival rates were >90% and increased by <1% per week thereafter until term [25], which is in line with our finding that this threshold is an important developmental stage for the preterm newborn.

The human fetal lung, like other crucial organs, has a developmental timeline that progresses from the embryonic period until birth. The pulmonary alveoli, the definitive units of gas exchange, and its supportive structures develop during late fetal and early postnatal life. Postnatally, the lungs continue to mature as alveolarization and microvascular maturation continue until a "complete" functional lung is achieved [26]. Abrupt discontinuation of lung development process (i.e., preterm birth) results in a premature and immature functional lung, commonly presenting as neonatal respiratory distress syndrome (RDS) and its later complication, bronchopulmonary dysplasia (BPD), with increased incidence and severity with decreasing gestational age [12,27]. The primary cause of RDS is deficiency of pulmonary surfactant, which is developmentally regulated and starts at around 20 weeks' gestation [28]. However, most alveolar surfactant is produced after about 30–32 weeks' gestation, and preterm infants born before then will probably develop RDS [29], as both a decrease in the quantity and quality of surfactant contributes to decreased surfactant activity, resulting in RDS. Importantly, the characteristic clinical course of RDS is observed less frequently because of interventions that reduce the risk of RDS, including the use of antenatal glucocorticoid therapy, early intubation for surfactant therapy, and/or respiratory support for the preterm neonate [30]. Nevertheless, RDS is very common in extremely and very preterm infants, and even those born between 30 and 34 weeks have a significant risk for acute respiratory disease, as reported in a Swedish study in which approximately 30% of the moderate to late preterm infants had this complication [31]. As a result, it is common for preterm infants, especially those born very preterm, to be exposed to high levels of oxygen for extended periods owing to respiratory insufficiency. It is now known from multiple animal studies that prolonged inhalation of high levels of oxygen can permanently alter lung development, especially the formation of alveoli [21,32,33]. Preterm infants are more susceptible to oxygen toxicity compared with term infants due to their more immature antioxidant enzyme systems [28,34]. Other than oxygen toxicity, preterm infants may also suffer injury caused by mechanical ventilation (volutrauma) [35–37]. For extremely preterm infants who receive mechanical ventilation, the risk of BPD is high [38]. Because of the strong evidence that aggressive mechanical ventilation plays a major role in the pathogenesis of BPD, management of preterm infants requiring respiratory support has moved towards initial noninvasive measures. However, despite the use of noninvasive respiratory support, up to 50 percent of extremely preterm infants are eventually intubated and mechanically ventilated [39]. Extended ventilatory support carries an increased risk not only for BPD but also for later airway problems such as asthma and chronic obstructive pulmonary disease (COPD) [40]. Looking at chronic respiratory morbidities, retrospective studies and meta-analyses found prematurity to be an important risk factor for childhood wheezing disorders, specifically asthma [41–43]. In a large Swedish study, children born extremely preterm had a four-times higher risk of asthma compared to those born at term [44]. Furthermore, studies of children and young adults born moderately to very preterm show persistent and significant lung function deficits [17] and reduced exercise capacity in those born very preterm [45], all of which imply the significant health consequences of prematurity. In light of the evidence regarding the lung prematurity at extremely and very preterm gestational ages, our results can be easily interpreted. Interestingly, our study provides similar results to an earlier study carried out by our group [46], which also found that children born before 32 weeks' gestation were at a significantly higher risk for infectious morbidity, including respiratory infections, once again reinforcing the thesis that a premature lung is more susceptible to respiratory morbidity later in life.

Our study found significant higher rates of intrauterine infection in children born preterm, specifically in the extremely preterm group. This factor is known to affect infants' lung function and health [47]. Hence, we included it in the Cox regression models and found that it did not change the results of the study. As expected, rates of induced labor were far less common in the extremely and very preterm groups but still reached around 10% of deliveries in these groups. This might have resulted from the much higher rate of intrauterine infections that forced the attending obstetricians to induce labor in these early gestational ages. The same may be hypothesized due to the increased rates of hypertensive disorders found in the extremely and very preterm groups, though to a much lesser extent. Compared to term deliveries, diabetes was also more common in women who delivered very and moderate to late preterm, although this was not the case for those who delivered extremely preterm (probably since the gestational age of extreme prematurity is set before the recommended gestational age for GDM screening). Nevertheless, we also included these variables in the Cox model to find the results were unchanged. Finally, as expected, cesarean delivery rates were also significantly higher in the extremely and very preterm group. As this mode of delivery is known to affect long-term respiratory morbidity of the offspring even at term [48], we also included this variable as a possible confounder in the multivariant model. Even after controlling for all these possible confounders, the Cox model shows that being born preterm carries a significant risk for long-term respiratory morbidity, which correlates to the severity of prematurity.

The strength of this study stems from its large cohort and the long-term follow-up on children born in a single tertiary medical center. Being the sole hospital in the Negev region, we were able to combine databases from the Obstetrics and Pediatric wards to match the data for the offspring, assuming that if the child required hospitalization, it would have occurred in our institute. Since the Negev region has enjoyed positive immigration rates for the last 2 decades, this assumption is plausible. Maternal and obstetrical information was recorded by obstetricians assessing the mothers' medical prenatal care records immediately following delivery. Prior to archiving, all records were also reviewed by trained medical secretaries for accuracy and completeness of the information. Naturally, human errors are inevitable, but considering the large cohort of patients, we assume these are very marginal and statistically insignificant.

This was a retrospective study and as such, it has inherent flaws that allowed us only to assume an association between exposure (prematurity) and outcome (long-term morbidity) and not a causative explanation. Furthermore, many other factors could have led to the increased risk of long-term respiratory morbidity, rather than prematurity alone. We acknowledge that our dataset lacks some important factors for children long-term respiratory prognosis such as the treatments provided during pregnancy, offspring hospitalization or other post-discharge medical care. An important limitation to fully interpreting our results is the lack of data regarding the use of antenatal corticosteroid therapy. Dozens of randomized trials have confirmed that a course of antenatal corticosteroid therapy administered to women at risk for preterm delivery reduced the incidence and severity of respiratory distress syndrome (RDS) and mortality in offspring [49]. However, since the use of antenatal corticosteroid therapy for preterm delivery was already well established during the study period, we assume most patients in our cohort who presented with preterm labor or were induced to deliver in early gestational ages received the treatment non-selectively. Another important limitation of this study is the difficulty to account for some postnatal variables such as socioeconomic status and environmental influences, which might affect offspring respiratory health [50]. Our long-term database is also based on hospitalization records, and as such it includes only cases that were severe enough to require in-hospital treatment. Milder cases of respiratory morbidity that were treated in ambulatory setting were out of our reach. However, we assume that our results are actually an underestimation of the true prevalence of long-term respiratory morbidity in extremely and very preterm infants. Finally, this study evaluated long-term morbidity of offspring until 18 years of age and did not include longer-term follow-ups into adulthood, as a longer-term follow-up was not in the scope of this study. More studies investigating the longer-term follow-up of respiratory-related morbidity of the offspring according to gestational age would help to shed some more light on the true prevalence of gestational-age-related respiratory diseases of the total population.

5. Conclusions

Although the respiratory morbidity of a preterm infant is well described in the literature, most studies reported the inverse relationship between morbidity and gestational age but could not point out the exact gestational age threshold after which long-term morbidity is reduced. Our study shows 30 weeks' gestation to be an important milestone that can serve obstetricians and neonatologist in further calculating the risk and counselling patients on the long-term respiratory morbidity of a preterm infant. Obstetricians may also use our data when considering the consequences of preterm induction of labor for patients presenting with pregnancy complications, as we have demonstrated the risk of respiratory morbidity by gestational age. Our data also provide some reassurance for pediatricians and patients in the study cohort of hospitalized patients with respiratory morbidity, as most morbidities investigated here were found at relatively low rates.

Supplementary Materials: The following supporting information can be downloaded at: https://www.mdpi.com/article/10.3390/jcm11030751/s1. Table S1: Respiratory morbidity ICD-9 codes.

Author Contributions: Conceptualization, E.S.; methodology, E.S., G.P and T.W.; validation, E.S., G.P., G.G. and T.W.; formal analysis, T.W.; data curation, E.S., G.P. and T.W.; writing—original draft preparation, G.G.; writing—review and editing, E.S., G.P. and T.W; supervision, E.S.; project administration, E.S. All authors have read and agreed to the published version of the manuscript.

Funding: This research received no external funding.

Institutional Review Board Statement: The study was conducted in accordance with the Declaration of Helsinki, and approved by the Institutional Review Board of Soroka University Medical Center (SUMC) (protocol code SOR-19-0357, date of approval 10 October 2019).

Informed Consent Statement: Patient consent was waived due to the retrospective design using anonymous coding.

Acknowledgments: The first and second authors equally contributed to the article. No honorarium, grant or other form of payment was given to anyone to produce the manuscript.

Conflicts of Interest: The authors declare no conflict of interest.

References

1. Blencowe, H.; Cousens, S.; Chou, D.; Oestergaard, M.; Say, L.; Moller, A.-B.; Kinney, M.; Lawn, J.; The Born Too Soon Preterm Birth Action Group. Born Too Soon: The global epidemiology of 15 million preterm births. *Reprod. Health* **2013**, *10* (Suppl. 1), S2. [CrossRef] [PubMed]
2. Ohana, O.; Wainstock, T.; Sheiner, E.; Leibson, T.; Pariente, G. Long-term digestive hospitalizations of premature infants (besides necrotizing enterocolitis): Is there a critical threshold? *Arch. Gynecol. Obstet.* **2021**, *304*, 1–9. [CrossRef] [PubMed]
3. Chawanpaiboon, S.; Vogel, J.P.; Moller, A.-B.; Lumbiganon, P.; Petzold, M.; Hogan, D.; Landoulsi, S.; Jampathong, N.; Kongwattanakul, K.; Laopaiboon, M.; et al. Global, regional, and national estimates of levels of preterm birth in 2014: A systematic review and modelling analysis. *Lancet Glob. Health* **2019**, *7*, e37–e46. [CrossRef]
4. Blencowe, H.; Cousens, S.; Oestergaard, M.Z.; Chou, D.; Moller, A.-B.; Narwal, R.; Adler, A.; Garcia, C.V.; Rohde, S.; Say, L.; et al. National, regional, and worldwide estimates of preterm birth rates in the year 2010 with time trends since 1990 for selected countries: A systematic analysis and implications. *Lancet* **2012**, *379*, 2162–2172. [CrossRef]
5. Ely, D.M.; Driscoll, A.K. Infant Mortality in the United States, 2017: Data from the Period Linked Birth/Infant Death File. *Natl. Vital. Stat. Rep.* **2019**, *68*, 1–20. [PubMed]
6. Tyson, J.E.; Parikh, N.; Langer, J.; Green, C.; Higgins, R.D. Intensive Care for Extreme Prematurity—Moving beyond Gestational Age. *N. Engl. J. Med.* **2008**, *358*, 1672–1681. [CrossRef]
7. Helenius, K.; Sjörs, G.; Shah, P.S.; Modi, N.; Reichman, B.; Morisaki, N.; Kusuda, S.; Lui, K.; Darlow, B.A.; Bassler, D.; et al. Survival in Very Preterm Infants: An International Comparison of 10 National Neonatal Networks. *Pediatrics* **2017**, *140*, e20171264. [CrossRef]
8. Alleman, B.W.; Bell, E.F.; Li, L.; Dagle, J.M.; Smith, P.B.; Ambalavanan, N.; Laughon, M.M.; Stoll, B.J.; Goldberg, R.N.; Carlo, W.A.; et al. Individual and Center-Level Factors Affecting Mortality Among Extremely Low Birth Weight Infants. *Pediatrics* **2013**, *132*, e175–e184. [CrossRef]
9. Corchia, C.; Ferrante, P.; Da Frè, M.; Di Lallo, D.; Gagliardi, L.; Carnielli, V.; Miniaci, S.; Piga, S.; Macagno, F.; Cuttini, M. Cause-Specific Mortality of Very Preterm Infants and Antenatal Events. *J. Pediatr.* **2013**, *162*, 1125–1132.e4. [CrossRef]
10. Chandrasekharan, P.; Lakshminrusimha, S.; Chowdhury, D.; Van Meurs, K.; Keszler, M.; Kirpalani, H.; Das, A.; Walsh, M.C.; McGowan, E.C.; Higgins, R.D.; et al. Early Hypoxic Respiratory Failure in Extreme Prematurity: Mortality and Neurodevelopmental Outcomes. *Pediatrics* **2020**, *146*, e20193318. [CrossRef]
11. Kajekar, R. Environmental factors and developmental outcomes in the lung. *Pharmacol. Ther.* **2007**, *114*, 129–145. [CrossRef] [PubMed]
12. Stoll, B.J.; Hansen, N.I.; Bell, E.F.; Shankaran, S.; Laptook, A.R.; Walsh, M.C.; Hale, E.C.; Newman, N.S.; Schibler, K.; Carlo, W.A.; et al. Neonatal Outcomes of Extremely Preterm Infants from the NICHD Neonatal Research Network. *Pediatrics* **2010**, *126*, 443–456. [CrossRef] [PubMed]

13. Coathup, V.; Boyle, E.; Carson, C.; Johnson, S.; Kurinzcuk, J.J.; Macfarlane, A.; Petrou, S.; Rivero-Arias, O.; Quigley, M.A. Gestational age and hospital admissions during childhood: Population based, record linkage study in England (TIGAR study). *BMJ* **2020**, *371*, m4075. [CrossRef] [PubMed]
14. Kuint, J.; Lerner-Geva, L.; Chodick, G.; Boyko, V.; Shalev, V.; Reichman, B.; Heymann, E.; Zangen, S.; Smolkin, T.; Mimouni, F.; et al. Rehospitalization Through Childhood and Adolescence: Association with Neonatal Morbidities in Infants of Very Low Birth Weight. *J. Pediatr.* **2017**, *188*, 135–141.e2. [CrossRef]
15. Bolton, C.E.; Stocks, J.; Hennessy, E.; Cockcroft, J.R.; Fawke, J.; Lum, S.; McEniery, C.M.; Wilkinson, I.B.; Marlow, N. The EPICure Study: Association between Hemodynamics and Lung Function at 11 Years after Extremely Preterm Birth. *J. Pediatr.* **2012**, *161*, 595–601.e2. [CrossRef]
16. Choukroun, M.-L.; Feghali, H.; Vautrat, S.; Marquant, F.; Nacka, F.; Leroy, V.; Demarquez, J.-L.; Fayon, M.J. Pulmonary outcome and its correlates in school-aged children born with a gestational age ≤ 32 weeks. *Respir. Med.* **2013**, *107*, 1966–1976. [CrossRef]
17. Thunqvist, P.; Tufvesson, E.; Bjermer, L.; Winberg, A.; Fellman, V.; Domellöf, M.; Melén, E.; Norman, M.; Hallberg, J. Lung function after extremely preterm birth-A population-based cohort study (EXPRESS). *Pediatr. Pulmonol.* **2018**, *53*, 64–72. [CrossRef]
18. Hafström, M.; Källén, K.; Serenius, F.; Maršál, K.; Rehn, E.; Drake, H.; Ådén, U.; Farooqi, A.; Thorngren-Jerneck, K.; Strömberg, B. Cerebral Palsy in Extremely Preterm Infants. *Pediatrics* **2018**, *141*, e20171433. [CrossRef]
19. Hirvonen, M.; Ojala, R.; Korhonen, P.; Haataja, P.; Eriksson, K.; Gissler, M.; Luukkaala, T.; Tammela, O. Cerebral Palsy Among Children Born Moderately and Late Preterm. *Pediatrics* **2014**, *134*, e1584–e1593. [CrossRef]
20. Stocks, J.; Hislop, A.; Sonnappa, S. Early lung development: Lifelong effect on respiratory health and disease. *Lancet Respir. Med.* **2013**, *1*, 728–742. [CrossRef]
21. Harding, R.; Maritz, G. Maternal and fetal origins of lung disease in adulthood. *Semin. Fetal Neonatal Med.* **2012**, *17*, 67–72. [CrossRef] [PubMed]
22. Fawke, J.; Lum, S.; Kirkby, J.; Hennessy, E.; Marlow, N.; Rowell, V.; Thomas, S.; Stocks, J. Lung function and respiratory symptoms at 11 years in children born extremely preterm: The EPICure study. *Am. J. Respir. Crit. Care Med.* **2010**, *182*, 237–245. [CrossRef] [PubMed]
23. Kotecha, S.J.; Watkins, W.J.; Paranjothy, S.; Dunstan, F.D.; Henderson, A.J.; Kotecha, S. Effect of late preterm birth on longitudinal lung spirometry in school age children and adolescents. *Thorax* **2011**, *67*, 54–61. [CrossRef] [PubMed]
24. Kotecha, S.J.; Dunstan, F.D.; Kotecha, S. Long term respiratory outcomes of late preterm-born infants. *Semin. Fetal Neonatal Med.* **2012**, *17*, 77–81. [CrossRef] [PubMed]
25. Copper, R.L.; Goldenberg, R.L.; Creasy, R.K.; DuBard, M.B.; Davis, R.O.; Entman, S.S.; Iams, J.D.; Cliver, S.P. A multicenter study of preterm birth weight and gestational age—Specific neonatal mortality. *Am. J. Obstet. Gynecol.* **1993**, *168*, 78–84. [CrossRef]
26. Schittny, J.C. Development of the lung. *Cell Tissue Res.* **2017**, *367*, 427–444. [CrossRef]
27. Laughon, M.; Allred, E.N.; Bose, C.; O'Shea, T.M.; Van Marter, L.J.; Ehrenkranz, R.A.; Leviton, A.; ELGAN study investigators. Patterns of Respiratory Disease During the First 2 Postnatal Weeks in Extremely Premature Infants. *Pediatrics* **2009**, *123*, 1124–1131. [CrossRef]
28. Frank, L.; Sosenko, I.R. Development of lung antioxidant enzyme system in late gestation: Possible implications for the prematurely born infant. *J. Pediatr.* **1987**, *110*, 9–14. [CrossRef]
29. Fraser, J.; Walls, M.; McGuire, W. Respiratory complications of preterm birth. *BMJ* **2004**, *329*, 962–965. [CrossRef]
30. Finer, N.; Leone, T. Oxygen saturation monitoring for the preterm infant: The evidence basis for current practice. *Pediatr. Res.* **2009**, *65*, 375–380. [CrossRef]
31. Altman, M.; Vanpee, M.; Cnattingius, S.; Norman, M. Neonatal Morbidity in Moderately Preterm Infants: A Swedish National Population-Based Study. *J. Pediatr.* **2011**, *158*, 239–244.e1. [CrossRef] [PubMed]
32. Yee, M.; White, R.J.; Awad, H.A.; Bates, W.A.; McGrath-Morrow, S.A.; O'Reilly, M.A. Neonatal Hyperoxia Causes Pulmonary Vascular Disease and Shortens Life Span in Aging Mice. *Am. J. Pathol.* **2011**, *178*, 2601–2610. [CrossRef] [PubMed]
33. Kunig, A.M.; Balasubramaniam, V.; Markham, N.E.; Morgan, D.; Montgomery, G.; Grover, T.R.; Abman, S.H. Recombinant human VEGF treatment enhances alveolarization after hyperoxic lung injury in neonatal rats. *Am. J. Physiol. Cell. Mol. Physiol.* **2005**, *289*, L529–L535. [CrossRef] [PubMed]
34. Georgeson, G.D.; Szőny, B.J.; Streitman, K.; Varga, I.S.; Kovács, A.; Kovács, L.; László, A. Antioxidant enzyme activities are decreased in preterm infants and in neonates born via caesarean section. *Eur. J. Obstet. Gynecol. Reprod. Biol.* **2002**, *103*, 136–139. [CrossRef]
35. Hernandez, L.A.; Peevy, K.J.; Moise, A.A.; Parker, J.C. Chest wall restriction limits high airway pressure-induced lung injury in young rabbits. *J. Appl. Physiol.* **1989**, *66*, 2364–2368. [CrossRef] [PubMed]
36. Carlton, D.P.; Cummings, J.J.; Scheerer, R.G.; Poulain, F.R.; Bland, R.D. Lung overexpansion increases pulmonary microvascular protein permeability in young lambs. *J. Appl. Physiol.* **1990**, *69*, 577–583. [CrossRef] [PubMed]
37. Björklund, L.J.; Ingimarsson, J.; Curstedt, T.; John, J.; Robertson, B.; Werner, O.; Vilstrup, C.T.; Bj, L.J. Manual Ventilation with a Few Large Breaths at Birth Compromises the Therapeutic Effect of Subsequent Surfactant Replacement in Immature Lambs. *Pediatr. Res.* **1997**, *42*, 348–355. [CrossRef] [PubMed]
38. Laughon, M.M.; Langer, J.C.; Bose, C.L.; Smith, P.B.; Ambalavanan, N.; Kennedy, K.A.; Stoll, B.J.; Buchter, S.; Laptook, A.R.; Ehrenkranz, R.A.; et al. Prediction of Bronchopulmonary Dysplasia by Postnatal Age in Extremely Premature Infants. *Am. J. Respir. Crit. Care Med.* **2011**, *183*, 1715–1722. [CrossRef] [PubMed]

39. Klingenberg, C.; Wheeler, K.I.; McCallion, N.; Morley, C.J.; Davis, P.G. Volume-targeted versus pressure-limited ventilation in neonates. *Cochrane Database Syst. Rev.* **2017**, *10*, CD003666. [CrossRef]
40. Speer, C.P.; Silverman, M. Issues relating to children born prematurely. *Eur. Respir. J. Suppl.* **1998**, *27*, 13s–16s.
41. Been, J.V.; Lugtenberg, M.J.; Smets, E.; Van Schayck, C.P.; Kramer, B.W.; Mommers, M.; Sheikh, A. Preterm Birth and Childhood Wheezing Disorders: A Systematic Review and Meta-Analysis. *PLoS Med.* **2014**, *11*, e1001596. [CrossRef] [PubMed]
42. Leps, C.; Carson, C.; QLeps, C.; Carson, C.; Quigley, M.A. Gestational age at birth and wheezing trajectories at 3–11 years. *Arch. Dis. Child.* **2018**, *103*, 1138–1144. [CrossRef] [PubMed]
43. Jaakkola, M.S.; Ahmed, P.; Ieromnimon, A.; Goepfert, P.; Laiou, E.; Quansah, R. Preterm delivery and asthma: A systematic review and meta-analysis. *J. Allergy Clin. Immunol.* **2006**, *118*, 823–830. [CrossRef] [PubMed]
44. Källén, B.; Finnström, O.; Nygren, K.G.; Otterblad Olausson, P. Association between preterm birth and intrauterine growth retardation and child asthma. *Eur. Respir. J.* **2013**, *41*, 671–676. [CrossRef]
45. Smith, L.J.; van Asperen, P.P.; McKay, K.O.; Selvadurai, H.; Fitzgerald, D.A. Reduced Exercise Capacity in Children Born Very Preterm. *Pediatrics* **2008**, *122*, e287–e293. [CrossRef]
46. Davidesko, S.; Wainstock, T.; Sheiner, E.; Pariente, G. Long-Term Infectious Morbidity of Premature Infants: Is There a Critical Threshold? *J. Clin. Med.* **2020**, *9*, 3008. [CrossRef]
47. Kallapur, S.G.; Ikegami, M. Physiological consequences of intrauterine insults. *Paediatr. Respir. Rev.* **2006**, *7*, 110–116. [CrossRef]
48. Baumfeld, Y.; Walfisch, A.; Wainstock, T.; Segal, I.; Sergienko, R.; Landau, D.; Sheiner, E. Elective cesarean delivery at term and the long-term risk for respiratory morbidity of the offspring. *Eur. J. Nucl. Med. Mol. Imaging* **2018**, *177*, 1653–1659. [CrossRef]
49. McGoldrick, E.; Stewart, F.; Parker, R.; Dalziel, S.R. Antenatal corticosteroids for accelerating fetal lung maturation for women at risk of preterm birth. *Cochrane Database Syst. Rev.* **2020**, *2021*, CD004454. [CrossRef]
50. Maritz, G.S.; Morley, C.; Harding, R. Early developmental origins of impaired lung structure and function. *Early Hum. Dev.* **2005**, *81*, 763–771. [CrossRef]

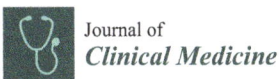

Article

Benefits of a Single Dose of Betamethasone in Imminent Preterm Labour

Natalia Saldaña-García [1,2,*], María Gracia Espinosa-Fernández [1], Celia Gómez-Robles [1], Antonio Javier Postigo-Jiménez [1], Nicholas Bello [1], Francisca Rius-Díaz [3] and Tomás Sánchez-Tamayo [1,4]

1. Department of Neonatology, Regional University Hospital of Malaga, 29010 Malaga, Spain; mgespinosaf@gmail.com (M.G.E.-F.); celiagr77@hotmail.com (C.G.-R.); ajpostigojimenez@gmail.com (A.J.P.-J.); nicholasbello90@gmail.com (N.B.); tomas.sanchez.tamayo@gmail.com (T.S.-T.)
2. School of Medicine, Malaga University, 29071 Malaga, Spain
3. Department of Preventive Medicine and Public Health, Biostatistics, School of Medicine, Malaga University, 29071 Malaga, Spain; rius@uma.es
4. Pediatrics Division, Malaga University, 29071 Malaga, Spain
* Correspondence: natalia@saldanagarcia.es

Abstract: Background: A complete course of prenatal corticosteroids reduces the possibility of morbimortality and neonatal respiratory distress syndrome (RDS). Occasionally, it is not possible to initiate or complete the maturation regimen, and the preterm neonate is born in a non-tertiary hospital. This study aimed to assess the effects of a single dose of betamethasone within 3 h before delivery on serious outcomes (mortality and serious sequelae) and RDS in preterm neonates born in tertiary vs. non-tertiary hospitals. Materials and methods: Preterm neonates who were <35 weeks and ≤1500 g, treated during a period of five years in a level IIIC NICU, were included in this retrospective cohort study. Participants were divided into groups as follows: NM, non-matured; PM, partial maturation (one dose of betamethasone up to 3 h antepartum). They were further divided based on their place of birth (NICU-IIIC vs. non-tertiary hospitals). The morbimortality rates and the severity of neonatal RDS were evaluated. Results: A total of 76 preterm neonates were included. A decrease in serious outcomes was found in the PM group in comparison to the NM group (OR = 0.2; 95%CI (0.07–0.9)), as well as reduced need for mechanical ventilation (54% vs. 68%). The mean time between maternal admission and birth was similar in both cohorts. The mean time from the administration of betamethasone to delivery was 1 h in the PM cohort. With regard to births in NICU-IIIC, the PM group performed better in terms of serious outcomes (32% vs. 45%) and the duration of mechanical ventilation (117.75 vs. 132.18 h) compared to the NM group. In neonates born in non-tertiary hospitals with PM in comparison to the NM group, a trend towards a reduced serious outcome (28.5% vs. 62.2%) and a decreased need for mechanical ventilation (OR = 0.09; 95%CI (0.01–0.8)) and maximum FiO_2 ($p = 0.01$) was observed. Conclusions: A single dose of betamethasone up to 3 h antepartum may reduce the rate of serious outcomes and the severity of neonatal RDS, especially in non-tertiary hospitals.

Keywords: antenatal corticosteroids; betamethasone; preterm infant; mortality; respiratory distress syndrome

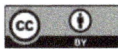

1. Introduction

The benefits of antenatal corticosteroid (ACS) administration in terms of reduced mortality and neonatal respiratory distress syndrome (RDS) rates in the preterm population are well documented in the scientific literature. Exposure to antenatal corticosteroid has also been associated with a decrease in the occurrence of intraventricular haemorrhage (IVH) [1].

These results have been verified for the full corticosteroid course, i.e., two doses of betamethasone, 12 mg each, 24 h apart, or four doses of dexamethasone, 6 mg each, 12 h apart, when preterm birth occurs within one to seven days of complete maturation [1–3].

With regard to precipitous preterm deliveries or situations that have imminent risk to the mother or foetus, at least one dose of antenatal corticosteroid is recommended, even if the completion of the course is not possible. However, on some occasions when a rapid birth is anticipated, the delivery may be completed without any prenatal corticosteroid dose [2,4].

The minimum time interval between the administration of antenatal corticosteroids and the appearance of significant beneficial effects for the preterm infant has not been determined. A mathematical estimate has recently been published in the EPICE study, which concludes that a single dose of corticosteroid administered 3 h before birth could lead to a decrease in mortality rate of up to 26% in the preterm population [5].

Situations regarding imminent delivery, either due to maternal, foetal, or membrane pathology, require rapid action by the obstetric team and may occur in both tertiary and secondary centres. Given the urgency of these events, on some occasions, it is not possible to transfer the pregnant woman from the regional hospital to the referral hospital, and the preterm is born in level I/II neonatal units, with subsequent transfer of the neonate, following stabilisation, to the referral level III unit for treatment [6].

The aim of this study was to assess the effects of a single dose of betamethasone administered within 3 h prior to birth with regard to serious outcomes and neonatal respiratory distress syndrome (RDS) in preterm infants born in tertiary vs. secondary hospitals.

2. Materials and Methods

A retrospective cohort study was conducted from 1 January 2015 to 31 December 2020, including preterm infants under 35 weeks of gestational age (GA), weighing ≤ 1500 g, admitted in a Neonatal Intensive Care Unit (NICU) IIIC level (Regional University Hospital of Málaga). Neonates with major malformations, genetic syndromes, and a prenatal diagnosis of intrauterine growth retardation were excluded from the study. Informed consent was obtained from parents upon admission to the NICU.

The study population was divided based on the course of lung maturation administered: non-matured (NM), which included preterm infants who received no antenatal corticosteroid dose, and partial maturation (PM), which included preterm infants who received a single dose of betamethasone (12 mg) within 3 h before birth.

The following variables were recorded as demographic and clinical characteristics: maternal age, primiparity, single/multiple gestations, the presence of gestational diabetes, hypertensive stages including pre-eclampsia, eclampsia and HELLP syndrome [7], chorioamnionitis [8,9] and third trimester haemorrhage (placental abruption, placenta praevia, uterine rupture, or vasa praevia). The following data were collected: place of birth, caesarean section, gestational age (GA) in weeks, anthropometric measurements at birth, gender, Apgar test score < 5 at 5 min of life and need for intubation at birth.

The main objective was to determine "serious outcomes", defined as death or survival with serious sequelae, which included the following: intraventricular haemorrhage grade III–IV (IVH), according to Papile classification [10]; periventricular leukomalacia (PVL) in either the cystic or non-cystic form, defined as changes in the signal intensity or echogenicity of the periventricular white matter, detected by ultrasound or MRI [11]; retinopathy of prematurity (ROP) requiring treatment [12]; necrotising enterocolitis (NEC) stage ≥ 2 according to the Bell classification [13]; moderate (the need for supplemental O_2 for ≥28 days and FiO_2 < 30% at 36 weeks postmenstrual age or discharge) or severe (the need for supplemental O_2 for ≥28 days greater than 30% and/or continuous positive pressure or mechanical ventilation at 36 weeks postmenstrual age or discharge) bronchopulmonary dysplasia (BPD) [14].

As secondary outcomes, the severity of RDS was determined by establishing the need for mechanical ventilation (MV), time on VM, maximum FiO_2 during admission, and the need for surfactant administration. Other variables analysed included hypotension during the first week of life requiring treatment (volume expansion or inotropic administration), persistent ductus arteriosus with haemodynamic repercussion requiring medical or surgical treatment, and the presence of sepsis (defined as clinical signs of sepsis and/or suggestive laboratory test results with a confirmatory blood culture), either early (in the first 72 h of life) or late (after the first 72 h of life) [15].

After the baseline characteristics of the study population were assessed, the population was further divided based on the place of birth (neonates born in the tertiary hospital with NICU-IIIC and neonates born in secondary hospitals and subsequently transferred to the NICU-IIIC).

Finally, in order to determine whether there would have at least been sufficient time to administer a dose in the non-matured (NM) group, the time elapsed from the admission of the pregnant woman to the emergency department to the birth of the preterm infant, in minutes, was analysed with regard to the PM and NM cohorts. This analysis was completed for the PM population using the time interval from maternal admission to prenatal corticosteroid administration and from prenatal corticosteroid administration to birth.

Contingency tables and the chi-squared test were used for the comparison of qualitative variables. In the 2 × 2 tables with a low number of observations ($n < 5$), Fisher's exact test and the odds ratios were calculated. To carry out pairwise comparisons of quantitative variables the Student's t-test was used. In all cases, a statistically significant difference was declared when the level for statistical significance was found to be below 5% ($p < 0.05$). For statistically significant results, a multivariate model was adjusted for the following confounding factors: GA, the presence of chorioamnionitis, hypertensive stages, and Apgar test score < 5 at 5 min of life. The statistical program SPSS 25.0 (IBM Corp., Armonk, NY, USA) was used.

This study was approved by the Provincial Ethics Committee of Málaga and by the Medical Management of the Regional University Hospital of Málaga.

3. Results

A total of 76 patients were studied, who were divided into the NM cohort ($n = 41$) and PM cohort ($n = 35$). The characteristics of the two cohorts are summarised in Table 1. The NM cohort had a higher percentage of secondary hospital births. The other variables, including GA, were distributed among the two cohorts without significant differences.

Table 1. Characteristics of the cohorts included in the study according to the maturation pattern.

	NM ($n = 41$)	PM ($n = 35$)	Significance (p) NM vs. PM *
Maternal age (years)	31.39 ± 7.06	30.55 ± 6.69	0.60
Primiparity	13 (38.2%)	11 (32.4%)	0.61
Multiple gestation	11 (26.8%)	7 (20%)	0.48
Gestational diabetes	2 (6.9%)	0	0.49
Hypertensive states	3 (7.7%)	1 (2.9%)	0.61
Chorioamnionitis	12 (30%)	9 (25.7%)	0.68
Third trimester haemorrhage	10 (25%)	6 (17.15%)	0.31
Secondary hospital birth	19 (46.3%)	7 (20%)	0.01
Caesarean section	26 (63.4%)	2 (65.7%)	0.92
Gestational age (weeks)	28.03 ± 2.61	27.84 ± 2.47	0.75
Birth weight (grams)	1040.98 ± 280.6	1025.9 ± 291.7	0.82
Height at birth (cm)	37.05 ± 3.1	35.7 ± 3.5	0.16
Head circumference at birth (cm)	26.65 ± 2.2	25.3 ± 2.8	0.08
Gender (female)	18 (43.9%)	20 (57.14%)	0.25
Apgar < 5 at 5 min	5 (14.3%)	2 (5.7%)	0.42
Intubation at birth	28 (68.3%)	20 (57.1%)	0.35

Qualitative variables are expressed as n (%); quantitative variables as mean ± standard deviation. * Fisher's exact test/chi-squared test for qualitative variables; Student's t-test for quantitative variables. NM, not matured; PM, partial maturation.

A comparison analysis between the NM versus PM cohort is shown in Table 2. The rate of serious outcomes was found to be lower among those who received a single dose of betamethasone within 3 h prior to birth (PM cohort) than in those who received none, both in the unadjusted and in the multivariable model (OR 0.2 95%CI (0.07–0.9)). Likewise, preterm infants who received a pre-birth dose showed lower percentage rates of periventricular leukomalacia (PVL) and treated ROP. Trends that favoured the PM cohort were found in relation to other outcome variables, which included: less need for MV, shorter MV times, lower maximum FiO_2 during admission, less hypotension requiring treatment during the first week of life, and reduced rates of moderate/severe BPD.

Table 2. Neonatal outcomes of cohort comparison according to maturation pattern.

	NM (n = 41)	PM (n = 35)	Significance (p) *	OR(95%CI) Unadjusted	OR(95%CI) Adjusted ‡
Exitus	6 (14.6%)	7 (20%)	0.53	1.4 (0.44–4.83)	
Serious outcome	22 (53.7%)	11 (31.4%)	0.05	0.3 (0.15–1)	0.2 (0.07–0.9)
Severe IVH	7 (17.1%)	5 (14.3%)	0.74	0.8 (0.2–2.8)	
PVL	5 (12.2%)	0	0.05	0.8 (0.7–0.9)	NA
NEC ≥ 2nd degree	1 (2.6%)	0	1	0.9 (0.92–1)	NA
Treated ROP	5 (12.2%)	0	0.05	0.8 (0.7–0.9)	NA
Arterial hypotension	17 (42.5%)	11 (31.4%)	0.32	0.6 (0.2–1.6)	
Treated PDA	14 (34.1%)	16 (45.7%)	0.42	1.6 (0.6–4.1)	
Moderate/severe BPD	10 (28.6%)	3 (10.7%)	0.11	0.3 (0.07–1.2)	
Surfactant requirement	33 (80.5%)	28 (80%)	0.95	0.9 (0.31–3)	
MV	28 (68.3%)	19 (54.4%)	0.21	0.5 (0.2–1.4)	
Early sepsis	2 (5.1%)	1 (2.9%)	1	0.5 (0.04–6.2)	
Late sepsis	14 (35.9%)	10 (28.6%)	0.62	0.7 (0.2–1.9)	
			Significance (p) †		
MV time (hours)	159.42 ± 176.51	98.84 ± 81.17	0.12		
Maximum FiO_2	50.12 ± 26.37	42.32 ± 24.77	0.19		

Variables are expressed as n (%) and mean ± standard deviation for qualitative and quantitative variables, respectively. * Fisher's exact test/chi-squared test; † Student's t-test. ‡ Results of multivariate analysis are shown for significant variables in the unadjusted model. NM, not matured; PM, partial maturation; IVH, intraventricular haemorrhage; PVL, periventricular leukomalacia; NEC, necrotising enterocolitis; ROP, retinopathy of prematurity; PDA, patent ductus arteriosus; BPD, bronchopulmonary dysplasia; MV, mechanical ventilation. NA, not applicable, as one of the cohorts analysed had a result of "0" for the variable.

Data concerning the time elapsed (in minutes) from the admission of the pregnant woman to preterm birth are shown in Figure 1. Surprisingly, somewhat longer periods of time elapsed with regard to the NM cohort, although the difference did not reach statistical significance (NM vs. PM, mean ± standard deviation: 150.7 ± 118.9 vs. 126.1 ± 57.5, respectively).

For the PM cohort, the time intervals from the admission of the pregnant woman to antenatal betamethasone administration and from corticosteroid administration to preterm birth were found to be 35.4 ± 58.2 and 61.8 ± 44.4 min, respectively.

An analysis of the NM and PM cohorts of preterm infants born at the tertiary hospital was performed (Table 3). In the analysis of NM versus PM, a trend towards lower serious outcome rates in the group receiving a single dose of antenatal corticosteroid was seen. Better results were also observed in terms of the rates of PVL, severe IVH, moderate/severe BPD, arterial hypotension in the first week of life, and the need for surfactant therapy, as well as with regard to MV time.

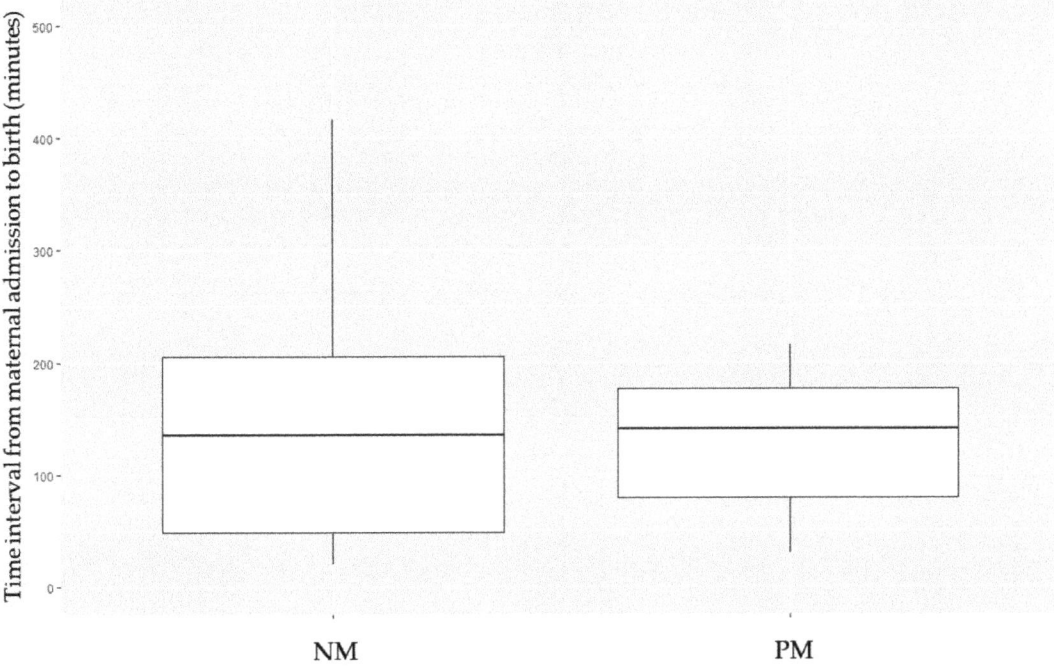

Figure 1. Time interval (in minutes) from the admission of the pregnant woman to the birth of the preterm neonate, depending on the maturation pattern received. NM, non-matured. PM, partial maturation.

Table 3. Comparison of the tertiary hospital birth population based on the maturation pattern received.

	NM (n = 22)	PM (n = 28)	Significance (p) *	OR (95%CI)
Exitus	5 (22.7%)	6 (21.4%)	0.91	0.9 (0.24–3.55)
Serious outcome	10 (45.5%)	9 (32.1%)	0.33	0.5 (0.18–1.80)
Severe IVH	3 (13.6%)	4 (14.2%)	1	1.2 (0.21–5.29)
PVL	2 (9.1%)	0	1	0.9 (0.79–1.03)
NEC ≥ 2nd degree	1 (5%)	0	0.41	0.9 (0.85–1.05)
Treated ROP	2 (9.1%)	0	0.18	0.9 (0.79–1.03)
Arterial hypotension	8 (38.1%)	9 (32.1%)	0.76	0.7 (0.23–2.51)
Treated PDA	6 (27.6%)	13 (46.3%)	0.16	2.3 (0.69–7.64)
Moderate/severe BPD	3 (17.6%)	3 (13.6%)	1	0.7 (0.12–4.21)
Surfactant requirement	18 (81.8%)	22 (78.5%)	0.77	0.8 (0.19–3.33)
MV	11 (50%)	16 (57.1%)	0.61	1.3 (0.43–4.09)
Early sepsis	1 (4.5%)	1 (3.5%)	1	0.7 (0.04–11.91)
Late sepsis	5 (22.7%)	9 (32.1%)	0.75	1.4 (00.39–5.14)
			(p) †	
MV time (hours)	132.18 ± 186.91	113.75 ± 79.82	0.76	
Maximum FiO$_2$	45.80 ± 27.96	45.92 ± 26.18	0.98	

Results are expressed as n (%) and mean ± standard deviation for qualitative and quantitative variables, respectively. * Fisher's exact test/chi-squared test; † Student's t-test. NM, non-matured; PM, partial maturation; CM, complete maturation; IVH, intraventricular haemorrhage; PVL, periventricular leukomalacia; NEC, necrotising enterocolitis; ROP, retinopathy of prematurity; PDA, patent ductus arteriosus; BPD, bronchopulmonary dysplasia; MV, mechanical ventilation.

The analysis of the effects of partial maturation in the secondary hospital population is shown in Table 4. The decrease in the number of cases had an impact on the statistical power of this comparison, although the trends towards better results in relation to the PM cohort with regard to the rates of serious outcomes and different morbidities (severe IVH, PVL, ROP, and arterial hypotension during the first week of life) were maintained. There was a significant decrease in the need for MV that favoured the PM cohort, which was maintained following adjustment for confounding factors (OR 0.09 95%CI (0.01–0.8)). The maximum FiO_2 during admission was significantly lower in the PM group, $p = 0.01$; 95%CI (−45.19, −5.63). Time on VM was also significantly lower in the PM group, but when it was adjusted for confounding factors, significance was lost ($p = 0.19$).

Table 4. Comparison of the secondary hospital birth population based on the maturation pattern received.

	NM (n = 19)	PM (n = 7)	Significance (p) *	OR (95%CI) Unadjusted	OR (95%CI) Adjusted ‡
Exitus	1 (5.3%)	1 (14.3%)	0.47	3 (0.16–55.72)	
Serious outcome	12 (62.2%)	2 (28.5%)	0.19	0.2 (0.03–1.5)	
Severe IVH	4 (21.1%)	1 (14.2%)	1	0.6 (0.05–6.8)	
PVL	3 (15.8%)	0	0.54	0.8 (0.6–1.02)	
NEC ≥ 2nd degree	0	0	-	-	-
Treated ROP	3 (15.8%)	0	0.54	0.8 (0.6–1.02)	
Arterial hypotension	9 (47.4%)	2 (28.5%)	0.65	0.4 (0.06–2.88)	
Treated PDA	8 (42.1%)	3 (42.8%)	1	1.03 (0.17–5.9)	
Moderate/severe BPD	7 (38.9%)	0	0.13	0.2 (0.02–2.09)	
Surfactant requirement	15 (78.9%)	6 (85.7%)	0.69	1.6 (0.14–17.1)	
MV	17 (89.5%)	3 (42.8%)	0.02	0.08 (0.01–0.71)	0.09 (0.01–0.8)
Early sepsis	1 (5.3%)	0	1	0.94 (0.85–1.05)	
Late sepsis	9 (47.4%)	1 (14.3%)	0.19	0.18 (0.02–1.84)	
			Significance (p) †		Adjusted significance (p) ‡
MV time (hours)	177.05 ± 172.92	19.33 ± 16.04	0.002		0.19
Maximum FiO_2	55.16 ± 24.17	28.42 ± 11.04	0.01		0.01

Variables are expressed as n (%) and mean ± standard deviation for qualitative and quantitative variables, respectively. * Fisher's exact test/chi-squared test; † Student's t-test. ‡ Results of multivariate analysis are shown for significant variables in the unadjusted model. NM, non-matured; PM, partial maturation; IVH, intraventricular haemorrhage; PVL, periventricular leukomalacia; NEC, necrotising enterocolitis; ROP, retinopathy of prematurity; PDA, patent ductus arteriosus; BPD, bronchopulmonary dysplasia; MV, mechanical ventilation.

A further analysis was performed to assess the effect of birth in secondary hospitals and the subsequent transfer of the preterm infant with regard to the non-matured and partially matured populations (Tables 5 and 6, respectively). The analysis of the NM group revealed worse results for the group born in the secondary hospital, with a significantly higher rate of the need for MV in both the unadjusted and confounder-adjusted models (OR 9.05 95%CI (1.62–50.62)). Comparison between the PM groups based on place of birth showed similar percentage rates of serious outcome and different morbidities. The tertiary hospital PM cohort had a longer MV time; however, when it was adjusted for confounding factors, this significance disappeared ($p = 0.46$; OR 0.38 95%CI (−126.6–9)).

Table 5. Comparison of the non-matured population by place of birth.

	NM_T (n = 22)	NM_S (n = 19)	Significance (p) *	OR (95%CI) Unadjusted	OR (95%CI) Adjusted ‡
Exitus	5 (22.7%)	1 (5.3%)	0.11	0.18 (0.02–1.78)	
Serious outcome	10 (45.5%)	12 (62.2%)	0.25	2.05 (0.58–7.21)	
Severe IVH	3 (13.6%)	4 (21.1%)	0.68	1.68 (0.32–8.73)	
PVL	2 (9.1%)	3 (15.8%)	0.64	1.87 (0.27–12.61)	
NEC ≥ 2nd degree	1 (5%)	0	1	0.95 (0.85–1.05)	
Treated ROP	2 (9.1%)	3 (15.8%)	0.64	1.87 (0.27–12.61)	
Arterial hypotension	8 (38.1%)	9 (47.4%)	0.55	1.46 (0.41–5.15)	
Treated PDA	6 (27.6%)	8 (42.1%)	0.31	1.93 (0.52–7.17)	
BPD	3 (17.6%)	7 (38.9%)	0.16	2.9 (0.62–14.22)	
Surfactant requirement	18 (81.8%)	15 (78.9%)	0.81	0.83 (0.17–3.91)	
MV	11 (50%)	17 (89.5%)	0.007	8.5 (1.57–45.91)	9.05 (1.62–50.62)
Early sepsis	1 (5%)	1 (5.3%)	0.97	1.05 (0.6–18.17)	
Late sepsis	5 (25%)	9 (47.4%)	0.14	2.7 (0.7–10.46)	
			Significance (p) †		
MV time (hours)	132.18 ± 186.91	177.05 ± 172.92	0.52		
Maximum FiO$_2$	45.8 ± 27.96	55.16 ± 24.17	0.27		

Variables are expressed as n (%) and mean ± standard deviation for qualitative and quantitative variables, respectively. * Fisher's exact test/chi-squared test; † Student's t-test. ‡ Results of multivariate analysis are shown for significant variables in the unadjusted model. NM_T, not-matured (tertiary hospital); NM_S, not-matured (secondary hospital); IVH, intraventricular haemorrhage; PVL, periventricular leukomalacia; NEC, necrotising enterocolitis; ROP, retinopathy of prematurity; PDA, patent ductus arteriosus; BPD, bronchopulmonary dysplasia; MV, mechanical ventilation.

Table 6. Comparison of the population with partial maturation by place of birth.

	PM_T (n = 28)	PM_S (n = 7)	Significance (p) *	OR (95%CI)
Exitus	6 (21.4%)	1 (14.3%)	1	0.61 (0.06–6.10)
Serious outcome	9 (32.1%)	2 (28.5%)	1	0.8 (0.13–5.22)
Severe IVH	4 (14.2%)	1 (14.2%)	1	1 (0.09–10.66)
PVL	0	0	-	-
NEC ≥ 2nd grade	0	0	-	-
Treated ROP	0	0	-	-
Arterial hypotension	9 (32.1%)	2 (28.5%)	1	0.8 (0.13–5.22)
Treated PDA	13 (46.3%)	3 (42.8%)	0.94	0.8 (0.16–4.6)
Moderate/severe BPD	3 (13.6%)	0	1	0.8 (0.73–1.02)
Surfactant requirement	22 (78.5%)	6 (85.7%)	0.64	1.6 (0.16–16.3)
MV	16 (57.1%)	3 (42.8%)	0.67	0.5 (0.1–2.9)
Early sepsis	1 (3.6%)	0	1	0.9 (0.89–1.03)
Late sepsis	9 (32.1%)	1 (14.3%)	0.64	0.3 (0.03–3.37)
			Significance (p) †	Adjusted significance (p) ‡
MV time (hours)	113.75 ± 79.82	19.33 ± 16.04	<0.01	0.46
Maximum FiO$_2$	45.92 ± 28.18	28.42 ± 11.04	0.09	0.12

Variables are expressed as n (%) and mean ± standard deviation for qualitative and quantitative variables, respectively. * Fisher's exact test/chi-squared test; † Student's t-test. ‡ Results of multivariate analysis are shown for significant variables in the unadjusted model. PM_T, partial maturation (tertiary hospital); PM_S, partial maturation (secondary hospital); IVH, intraventricular haemorrhage; PVL, periventricular leukomalacia; NEC, necrotising enterocolitis; ROP, retinopathy of prematurity; PDA, patent ductus arteriosus; BPD, bronchopulmonary dysplasia; MV, mechanical ventilation.

4. Discussion

The time interval between the administration of antenatal corticosteroid and preterm birth is of utmost importance, as the beneficial effects of corticosteroids on the rates of serious outcomes and respiratory distress depend on this interval [3,16–18].

There are clinical situations where prenatal corticosteroid therapy is not initiated because birth is considered imminent, or the full course cannot be completed. Additionally, in these high-risk situations, the cascade of events prevents the transfer of the pregnant woman if she is in a non-tertiary hospital, and the premature birth takes place in a level I/II neonatal unit [6,19].

Our results show a 22.3% decrease in serious outcomes in favour of the group that received a single dose of betamethasone immediately before birth, which is in line with the results found in the literature [5,16]. In the EPICE study published by Norman et al. (2017), a mathematical estimate was made based on the results obtained from a cohort of 4594 preterm infants, concluding that a single dose of corticosteroid administered within 3 h before birth could reduce the mortality rate associated with non-matured neonates up to 26% [5]. In our study, we found no significant differences in mortality rates, probably due to insufficient sample size (289 infants in each arm would have been needed to obtain sufficient power to detect a 20% decrease in mortality). The minimum time interval between prenatal corticosteroid administration and preterm birth to obtain the benefits of lung maturation has not been determined. In our study, with a mean of 61.8 ± 44.4 min between the administration of a single dose of corticosteroid and preterm birth and up to a maximum of 3 h, better results were found for the PM cohort.

In animal models, betamethasone levels that are effective for lung maturation (1–4 ng/mL) have been detected in the umbilical cord at the time of prenatal administration. [20] Based on these models, it was determined that in pregnant women > 28 weeks, the intramuscular administration of 11.4 mg of betamethasone produces levels > 1 ng/mL in the umbilical cord from the first hour of administration and are maintained for up to 1.4 days. Levels below 1 ng/mL increase the risk of surfactant therapy [21]. The placental transfer of betamethasone has been compared in single gestational, twin, and obese mothers, with no differences and levels > 1 ng/mL after the first dose of betamethasone [22]. These findings may support the biological plausibility of our results, although further studies are needed to analyse betamethasone levels in the umbilical cord after administration close to delivery.

In some situations where delivery is imminent, prenatal corticosteroids were not administered because it was considered that there would not be enough time for them to have an effect on the neonate. In our study, the timeline from the moment a pregnant woman was admitted to the emergency department to the birth of a preterm infant was recorded. This time interval was similar for non-matured and partially matured neonates (with a mean of 150 min for the NM group vs. 126 min for the PM group). Our results indicate that some of the preterm infants in the non-matured cohort could have benefited from the effects of a single dose of antenatal betamethasone.

Regarding the results found in preterm infants born in non-tertiary hospitals, the beneficial effect of antenatal betamethasone was evident. The PM cohort was found to exhibit a trend towards lower serious outcome rates. In addition, there was less need for MV and lower maximum FiO_2 in the group that received prenatal corticosteroids, although the sample of preterm infants for the PM cohort was smaller. In our study, a pre-delivery dose of betamethasone was shown to improve the outcome of preterm infants who had to undergo inter-hospital transfer to continue their treatment [19].

Mixed analysis between NM and PM cohorts born in secondary hospitals and the tertiary hospital reinforces the recommendations that favour preterm birth to take place in specialised units [6,19].

The strengths of this study include the homogeneity of the cohorts in terms of gestational age, birth weight, and perinatal history. Subsequent analysis controlling for confounding factors consolidated the results. The biological plausibility and the results according to the literature, support this research.

Several limitations of our study have to be pointed out. First, the retrospective approach of this research prevents from obtaining definitive conclusions about single-dose maturation, although it poses an important hypothesys to be tested in a larger prospective clinical trial. Second, the small sample size of the study population probably had an influence on not reaching significant differences in some of the variables analysed. Despite this, trends towards better results were observed in the group that received at least one dose. Finally, long-term outcomes have not been addressed in our study.

Given the international recommendation to initiate maturation with prenatal corticosteroids in situations of preterm birth, there are few cases in which maturation is not administered or in which it is administered just before delivery [23]. Further studies are necessary to confirm our results and determine the minimum time it takes for benefits from prenatal corticosteroid to be obtained by premature infants.

5. Conclusions

In conclusion, the administration of a single dose of betamethasone within 3 h prior to preterm birth may decrease the rates of serious outcomes and other morbidities in neonates. In particular, beneficial effects were observed when delivery takes place in non-tertiary hospitals. Given the available scientific evidence and the results of this study, we consider that urgent administration of antenatal betamethasone may be a safe and effective strategy in cases of imminent preterm birth.

Author Contributions: Conceptualisation, N.S.-G., T.S.-T. and C.G.-R.; methodology, M.G.E.-F. and F.R.-D.; software, N.S.-G.; validation, M.G.E.-F., T.S.-T. and C.G.-R.; formal analysis, N.S.-G., N.B.; investigation, N.S.-G., N.B. and A.J.P.-J.; resources, N.S.-G. and A.J.P.-J.; writing—original draft preparation, N.S.-G.; writing—review and editing, N.S.-G., T.S.-T., M.G.E.-F. All authors have read and agreed to the published version of the manuscript.

Funding: This research received no external funding.

Institutional Review Board Statement: The study was conducted according to the guidelines of the Declaration of Helsinki and approved by the Provincial Ethics Committee of Málaga and the Medical Management of the Regional University Hospital of Málaga (protocol code TD-CTR; date of approval 11 November 2020).

Informed Consent Statement: Informed consent was obtained from all subjects involved in the study.

Data Availability Statement: The data presented in this study are available on request from the corresponding author. The data are not publicly available due to data protection policies.

Conflicts of Interest: The authors declare no conflict of interest.

References

1. McGoldrick, E.; Stewart, F.; Parker, R.; Dalziel, S. Antenatal corticosteroids for accelerating fetal lung maturation for women at risk of preterm birth. *Cochrane Database Syst Rev.* **2020**, *12*, Cd004454.
2. Committee on Obstetric Practice. Committee Opinion No. 713: Antenatal Corticosteroid Therapy for Fetal Maturation. *Obstet Gynecol.* **2017**, *130*, e102–e109.
3. Lau, H.C.Q.; Tung, J.S.Z.; Wong, T.T.C.; Tan, P.L.; Tagore, S. Timing of antenatal steroids exposure and its effects on neonates. *Arch Gynecol Obstet.* **2017**, *296*, 1091–1096. [CrossRef] [PubMed]
4. Briceno-Perez, C.; Reyna-Villasmil, E.; Vigil-De-Gracia, P. Antenatal corticosteroid therapy: Historical and scientific basis to improve preterm birth management. *Eur. J. Obstet Gynecol. Reprod. Biol.* **2019**, *234*, 32–37. [CrossRef]
5. Norman, M.; Piedvache, A.; Børch, K.; Huusom, L.D.; Bonamy, A.E.; Howell, E.A.; Jarreau, P.-H.; Maier, R.F.; Pryds, O.; Toome, L.; et al. Association of Short Antenatal Corticosteroid Administration-to-Birth Intervals With Survival and Morbidity Among Very Preterm Infants: Results From the EPICE Cohort. *JAMA Pediatr.* **2017**, *171*, 678–686. [CrossRef]
6. Rite Gracia, S.; Fernández Lorenzo, J.R.; Echániz Urcelay, I.; Botet Mussons, F.; Herranz Carrillo, G.; Moreno Hernando, J.; Salguero, G.E.; Sánchez, L.M. Comité de Estándares y la Junta Directiva de la Sociedad Espanola de Neonatología. Health care levels and minimum recommendations for neonatal care. *An Pediatr.* **2013**, *79*, 51.e1–51.e11.
7. Gestational Hypertension and Preeclampsia: ACOG Practice Bulletin, Number 222. *Obstet Gynecol.* **2020**, *135*, e237–e260. [CrossRef]
8. Peng, C.C.; Chang, J.H.; Lin, H.Y.; Cheng, P.J.; Su, B.H. Intrauterine inflammation, infection, or both (Triple I): A new concept for chorioamnionitis. *Pediatr. Neonatol.* **2018**, *59*, 231–237. [CrossRef]
9. Committee on Obstetric Practice. Committee Opinion No. 712: Intrapartum Management of Intraamniotic Infection. *Obstet Gynecol.* **2017**, *130*, e95–e101.

10. Papile, L.A.; Burstein, J.; Burstein, R.; Koffler, H. Incidence and evolution of subependymal and intraventricular hemorrhage: A study of infants with birth weights less than 1500 gm. *J. Pediatr.* **1978**, *92*, 529–534. [CrossRef]
11. Gotardo, J.W.; Volkmer, N.F.V.; Stangler, G.P.; Dornelles, A.D.; Bohrer, B.B.A.; Carvalho, C.G. Impact of peri-intraventricular haemorrhage and periventricular leukomalacia in the neurodevelopment of preterms: A systematic review and meta-analysis. *PLoS ONE* **2019**, *14*, e0223427. [CrossRef]
12. Castro Conde, J.R.; Echániz Urcelay, I.; Botet Mussons, F.; Pallás Alonso, C.R.; Narbona, E.; Sánchez Luna, M. Retinopathy of prematurity. Prevention, screening and treatment guidelines. *An Pediatr.* **2009**, *71*, 514–523. [CrossRef]
13. Battersby, C.; Santhalingam, T.; Costeloe, K.; Modi, N. Incidence of neonatal necrotising enterocolitis in high-income countries: A systematic review. *Arch. Dis. Child. Fetal Neonatal Ed.* **2018**, *103*, F182–F189. [CrossRef]
14. Sánchez Luna, M.; Moreno Hernando, J.; Botet Mussons, F.; Fernández Lorenzo, J.R.; Herranz Carrillo, G.; Rite Gracia, S.; Salguero, G.E.; Echaniz, U.I. Bronchopulmonary dysplasia: Definitions and classifications. *An Pediatr.* **2013**, *79*, 262.e1–262.e6. [CrossRef]
15. Moro Serrano, M.; Fernández Pérez, C.; Figueras Alloy, J.; Pérez Rodríguez, J.; Coll, E.; Doménech Martínez, E.; Jiménez, R.; Pérez Sheriff, V.; Quero, J.J.; Serradilla, V.R.; et al. SEN1500: Design and implementation of a registry of infants weighing less than 1500 g at birth in Spain. *An Pediatr.* **2008**, *68*, 181–188. [CrossRef]
16. Travers, C.P.; Carlo, W.A.; McDonald, S.A.; Das, A.; Bell, E.F.; Ambalavanan, N.; Jobe, A.H.; Goldberg, R.N.; D'Angio, C.T.; Stoll, B.J.; et al. Mortality and pulmonary outcomes of extremely preterm infants exposed to antenatal corticosteroids. *Am. J. Obstet. Gynecol.* **2018**, *218*, 130.e1–130.e13. [CrossRef]
17. Norberg, H.; Kowalski, J.; Maršál, K.; Norman, M. Timing of antenatal corticosteroid administration and survival in extremely preterm infants: A national population-based cohort study. *BJOG Int. J. Obstet. Gynecol.* **2017**, *124*, 1567–1574. [CrossRef]
18. Battarbee, A.N.; Ros, S.T.; Esplin, M.S.; Biggio, J.; Bukowski, R.; Parry, S.; Zhang, H.; Huang, H.; Andrews, W.; Saade, G.; et al. Optimal timing of antenatal corticosteroid administration and preterm neonatal and early childhood outcomes. *Am. J. Obstet. Gynecol. MFM* **2020**, *2*, 100077. [CrossRef]
19. Moreno Hernando, J.; Thió Lluch, M.; Salguero García, E.; Rite Gracia, S.; Fernández Lorenzo, J.R.; Echaniz, U.I.; Botet, M.F.; Herranz, C.G.; Sánchez, L.M.; Comisión de Estándares de la Sociedad Española de Neonatología. Recommendations for neonatal transport. *An Pediatr.* **2013**, *79*, 117.e1–117.e7. [CrossRef]
20. Jobe, A.H.; Kemp, M.; Schmidt, A.; Takahashi, T.; Newnham, J.; Milad, M. Antenatal corticosteroids: A reappraisal of the drug formulation and dose. *Pediatr. Res.* **2021**, *89*, 318–325. [CrossRef]
21. Foissac, F.; Zheng, Y.; Hirt, D.; Lui, G.; Bouazza, N.; Ville, Y.; Goffinet, F.; Rozenberg, P.; Kayem, G.; Mandelbrot, L.; et al. Maternal Betamethasone for Prevention of Respiratory Distress Syndrome in Neonates: Population Pharmacokinetic and Pharmacodynamic Approach. *Clin. Pharmacol. Ther.* **2020**, *108*, 1026–1035. [CrossRef] [PubMed]
22. Gyamfi, C.; Mele, L.; Wapner, R.J.; Spong, C.Y.; Peaceman, A.; Sorokin, Y.; Dudley, D.J.; Johnson, F.; Leveno, K.J.; Caritis, S.N.; et al. The effect of plurality and obesity on betamethasone concentrations in women at risk for preterm delivery. *Am. J. Obstet. Gynecol.* **2010**, *203*, 219.e1–219.e5. [CrossRef]
23. Skoll, A.; Boutin, A.; Bujold, E.; Burrows, J.; Crane, J.; Geary, M.; Jain, V.; Liauw, J.; Mundle, W.; Murphy, K.; et al. No. 364-Antenatal Corticosteroid Therapy for Improving Neonatal Outcomes. *J. Obstet. Gynaecol. Can.* **2018**, *40*, 1219–1239. [CrossRef] [PubMed]

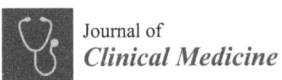

Article

Elastography and Metalloproteinases in Patients at High Risk of Preterm Labor

Izabela Dymanowska-Dyjak, Aleksandra Stupak *, Adrianna Kondracka, Tomasz Gęca, Arkadiusz Krzyżanowski and Anna Kwaśniewska

Department of Obstetrics and Pathology of Pregnancy, Medical University of Lublin, 20-081 Lublin, Poland; izabela.dyjak@gmail.com (I.D.-D.); adriannakondracka@wp.pl (A.K.); tomasz.geca@umlub.pl (T.G.); a_r_krzyzanowski@tlen.pl (A.K.); haniakwasniewska@gmail.com (A.K.)
* Correspondence: aleksandra.stupak@umlub.pl

Abstract: Preterm birth (PTB) is the leading cause of perinatal morbidity and mortality. Its etiopathology is multifactorial; therefore, many of the tests contain the assessment of the biochemical factors and ultrasound evaluation of the cervix in patients at risk of preterm delivery. The study aimed at evaluating the socioeconomic data, ultrasound examinations with elastography, plasma concentrations of MMP-8 and MMP-9 metalloproteinases, and vaginal secretions in the control group as well as patients with threatened preterm delivery (high-risk patients). The study included 88 patients hospitalized in the Department of Obstetrics and Pregnancy Pathology, SPSK 1, in Lublin. Patients were qualified to the study group (50) with a transvaginal ultrasonography of cervical length (CL) ≤ 25 mm. The control group (38) were patients with a physiological course of pregnancy with CL > 25 mm. In the study group, the median length of the cervix was 17.49 mm. Elastographic parameters: strain and ratio were 0.20 and 0.83. In the control group, the median length of the cervix was 34.73 mm, while the strain and ratio were 0.20 and 1.23. In the study group, the concentration of MMP-8 in the serum and secretions of the cervix was on average 74.17 and 155.46 ng/mL, but in the control group, it was significantly lower, on average 58.49 and 94.19 ng/mL. The concentration of MMP-9 in both groups was on the same level. Evaluation of the cervical length and measurement of MMP-8 concentration are the methods of predicting preterm delivery in high-risk patients. The use of static elastography did not meet the criteria of a PTB marker.

Keywords: preterm labor; high-risk patients; ultrasound; elastography; metalloproteinases; MMP-8; MMP-9

Citation: Dymanowska-Dyjak, I.; Stupak, A.; Kondracka, A.; Gęca, T.; Krzyżanowski, A ; Kwaśniewska, A. Elastography and Metalloproteinases in Patients at High Risk of Preterm Labor. *J. Clin. Med.* **2021**, *10*, 3886. https://doi.org/10.3390/jcm10173886

Academic Editor: Eyal Sheiner

Received: 4 July 2021
Accepted: 25 August 2021
Published: 29 August 2021

Publisher's Note: MDPI stays neutral with regard to jurisdictional claims in published maps and institutional affiliations.

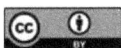

Copyright: © 2021 by the authors. Licensee MDPI, Basel, Switzerland. This article is an open access article distributed under the terms and conditions of the Creative Commons Attribution (CC BY) license (https://creativecommons.org/licenses/by/4.0/).

1. Introduction

Premature birth is a crucial issue of modern perinatology. According to the World Health Organization, it is estimated that approximately 15 million children are born prematurely. One million of them die due to complications related to prematurity, and a large proportion has physical and mental disabilities [1]. In Poland, the percentage of premature births is close to the European average and amounts to approximately 6.7% of all live births (i.e., approximately 27,000 children).

Preterm births have increased in the last 20 years. It results, inter alia, from a delay in the reproductive age of women giving birth for the first time and, therefore, a greater number of maternal health problems, such as diabetes, hypertension, infertility treatment, cancer [1]. The same data indicate a higher survival rate of premature babies, which is inextricably linked with an improvement in neonatal care in most countries. Currently, about 90% of babies born at 28 weeks of pregnancy have a chance of survival. Research conducted in Great Britain shows that the survival rate of newborns in the group between 22 and 23 weeks of gestation is approximately 51%, in 24 weeks of pregnancy—47%, and in 25 weeks—67% and half of the newborns born after 25 weeks of pregnancy develop normally [2]. The definition of preterm labor includes the criterion of the duration of pregnancy, and it is delivery after the 22nd week of pregnancy and before the 37th week of pregnancy [1].

The greatest risk of complications concerns children born up to the 33rd week of pregnancy. Therefore, it is important to identify risk factors for preterm labor, and thus qualify pregnant women to the group at risk of premature delivery [3]. These patients can be divided into two groups:

- High-risk group (these are patients who have had a history of preterm labor in previous pregnancies—about 15% of all preterm births).
- Low-risk group (85% of preterm deliveries without burdened medical history).

Preterm labor risk factors can be divided into maternal, environmental, occupational, and obstetric factors.

The maternal factors include:

- Low socioeconomic status;
- Black race (compared to the white race) [4];
- Low level of education;
- Age below 18 and over 40 [5];
- Free marital status;
- Low maternal body weight before pregnancy (BMI below 19) [6];
- Thyroid diseases and other maternal diseases, such as urinary tract infections and periodontal diseases [7].

The environmental and professional factors include:

- Environment pollution;
- Smoking and drugs addiction;
- Stress (doubling the risk of preterm labor) [8];
- Hard physical work, shift work, night work, and long-term standing [9].

The obstetric factors include:

- A history of preterm labor;
- Multiple pregnancies;
- Bleeding from the genital tract [10];
- Intrauterine infection;
- Endometriosis [11];
- Hypertension and diabetes;
- Incorrect amount of amniotic fluid;
- Abdominal surgery in the second and third trimesters of pregnancy.

The etiology of preterm labor is multifactorial. About 50% of premature deliveries are associated with spontaneous uterine contractions; in 20–30% of cases, it is the premature termination of pregnancy due to medical indications, while 20% of them are caused by the preterm premature rupture of membranes (PPROM). Romero, in 2006, proposed the so-called "common way of delivery", which involves the activation of multiple systems that lead to biochemical and anatomical changes aimed at the expulsion of the fetus and postpartum [12]. According to the current state of knowledge, infections are the main cause of premature births. It is assumed that they are responsible for about 40% of premature births. The pathogens identified in the amniotic fluid include both aerobic and anaerobic bacteria and viruses. The cytokines involved in the activation of the "common pathway" in preterm labor are IL-1 and TNF-alpha. It has been shown that the concentration of IL-1 and IL-8 in the cervicovaginal secretion is significantly higher in women who gave birth prematurely [13]. In addition, IL-1 stimulates the production of prostaglandins by the temporal and amniotic fluid, thereby inducing uterine contractile activity. In the case of TNF-alpha, there are reports that the concentration of this substance is much higher in patients whose preterm labor is caused by rupture of the membranes [14]. It is related to the stimulation of the production of metalloproteinases, mainly MMP-1, MMP-2, and MMP-9, which, etiopathogenetically, are associated with premature rupture of the fetal bladder and maturation of the cervix [15]. Metalloproteinases are enzymes that catalyze the degradation processes of collagen types I, II, III, IV, VII, X, and elastin. Their activity in the membranes of the fetus is regulated by many different substances, including trypsin, elastase, and thrombin. Anti-inflammatory cytokines, such as IL-10, also play an important role in the mechanism that induces preterm labor and are involved in the immune recognition and maintenance of pregnancy.

The causes of preterm labor also include cervical insufficiency, which we define as painless opening and shortening of the cervix. The risk of premature childbirth is estimated at 75% when the assessment of the length of the cervix is below 25 mm in pregnant women before the 20th week of pregnancy [16]. There are also biochemical indicators of preterm labor; these include fetal fibronectin.

Ultrasound is one of the best methods of assessing the length of the cervical canal. During ultrasound examination of the cervix, the following parameters should be taken into account:

- Measurement of the length of the cervical canal;
- Assessment of the shape of the internal os and the cervical canal;
- Measurement of the internal os;
- Measurement of the length of the invagination of the fetal bladder;
- Cervical index;
- Assessment of the posterior angle of the cervix.

The total length of the cervix is the distance between the inner and outer os. Its functional length is the distance between the lower pole of the amniotic sac, to the cervix, and the external os. In practice, functional length assessment is important for the prediction of preterm labor. We use the TYVU (Trust Your Vaginal Ultrasound) scheme to evaluate the shape of the internal os. Incorrect values of the index for patients from the higher risk group significantly increase the real risk of preterm labor. According to the Fetal Medicine Foundation (FMF), in order to correctly assess the length of the cervical canal, certain conditions must be met [17]. The elastography technique was first described in 1991 by Ophir and his colleagues [18]. It is a method of imaging organs and tissues, assessing their stiffness and hardness. It determines the susceptibility of the examined tissue to compression and mechanical decompression. This is possible thanks to digital ultrasound and appropriate image processing obtained with a volumetric probe. Currently, the most advanced variant of this method is dynamic elastography (in other words, Shear Wave Elastography). It is based on the objective assessment and measurement of the stiffness of the tissue to obtain its numerical value expressed in kPa or m/s using the supersonic effect in the Mach cone and Young's modulus (on the extensibility and compressibility of the media) [19].

Elastography is a modern diagnostic method that is based on the fact that the hardness of the tissue/organ changes significantly as a result of the disease process. There are attempts to predict preterm labor by assessment of placental flexibility. The rectus abdominis muscle and the subcutaneous tissue were used as reference points for the stiffness coefficients. In the case of the second factor, its value measured in the second trimester of pregnancy can be effectively used as a marker of preterm labor [20]. Metalloproteinases (MMPs) are proteolytic enzymes that contain a zinc ion in the catalytic center. Both the MMP-8 and MMP-9 enzymes are of crucial importance during labor. MMP-9 has also been identified in the amniotic fluid in patients at risk of preterm labor and in delivery patients [21]. There are reports on the relationship between ultrasound examination and the assessment of the concentration of MMP-9 as a marker of preterm labor within 7 days from the examination. Most importantly, the concentration of MMP-9 in the maternal blood plasma remains stable during uncomplicated preterm pregnancy until the onset of full-term labor. In active preterm labor, the concentration of MMP-9 is increased in the amniotic fluid. MMP-9 is concentrated and activated in the amniotic fluid during pregnancy complicated by premature rupture of the membranes. Moreover, in the case of inflammation of the membranes and PROM, the expression of the gene encoding MMP-9 is increased. Assuming a cut-off value of 15 mm for the measurement of the cervical length and a proMMP-9 concentration of 67.157 ng/mL in plasma, we can achieve similarly negative predictive values for preterm labor, approx. 96% for the length of the cervix and 96% for the concentration of pro-MMP-9, while for positive predictors, 69% and 60% respectively. Interestingly, when both prognostic factors were combined, the sensitivity and specificity of the test improved. However, in order to be able to use the combination of both tests to predict premature labor, studies on a larger group of patients are needed [15]. Increased concentration of MMP-8 is not only associated with the maturation of the cervix during labor but also in preterm labor, PPROM, and intrauterine infection. Increased concentrations of MMP-8 in the blood serum are associated with an increase in the number of leukocytes in vaginal swabs [22]. Neutrophils and the concentration of MMP-8 in the amniotic fluid are believed to be an inflammatory response to ascending vaginal infections [7,12,23–25].

As shown, preterm labor is a complex problem, and its diagnosis is one of the most important obstetric issues.

2. The Aim of the Study

The aim of this study was a biochemical and ultrasound evaluation of the cervix in patients at high-risk of preterm labor.

The aim of the work was achieved by assessing:

- Socioeconomic data;
- Ultrasound examinations with elastography;
- The concentration of MMP-8 and MMP-9 metalloproteinases in plasma and in vaginal secretions in the group of patients at risk of preterm labor compared to the control group of pregnant women with a physiological course of pregnancy.

3. Material and Methods

The clinical material of the study included 88 pregnant women hospitalized at the Department of Obstetrics and Pathology of Pregnancy of the Medical University of Lublin. Patients who met the criteria for high-risk premature labor between 25 and 38 weeks gestation qualified for the study group. The control group consisted of patients who did not report premature delivery symptoms without concomitant diseases. After learning about the purpose and method of conducting the research, all patients gave their informed and written consent to participate in this project. The consent for the research was issued by the Bioethics Committee at the Medical University of Lublin (KE-0254/134/2009 and KE-0254/294/2017).

In patients hospitalized at the Department of Obstetrics and Pathology of Pregnancy at the Medical University of Lublin with symptoms of premature labor, the diagnostic standard is an ultrasound examination, in which, in addition to the assessment of the fetal biometry and anatomy, the length of the cervix was determined. Blood samples were also collected from the patients included in the study, and a swab was taken from the posterior vaginal fornix during the gynecological examination preceding the ultrasound examination. The VolusonTM E8 with Elastography Analysis mode was used for the ultrasound examination. An endovaginal ultrasound was performed using an endoscopic probe (VolusonTM E8, RIC5-9-D). During the examination, the patients were asked to assume the lithotomy position. An endovaginal probe was placed in the anterior vaginal fornix, and the bladder was identified as an orientation point. A standard sagittal image of the cervix was then obtained, and the length of the cervix was measured. The probe, with elastography mode on, was used to produce up to five compression and decompression cycles. After confirming the correct compression and manual decompression in the form of a green quality bar in the lower-left corner of the screen, a measurement was made with each cycle lasting about 1 s. During each cycle, a tissue shift of approximately 1 cm was achieved. On the images obtained in this way, two regions were selected: area A on the upper cervical lip and area B on the bones of the fetal skull as the hardest reference point. Within these areas, circles of 5 mm in diameter were placed. From these circles, the Elastography Analysis program computed numerical values for the strain ratio and SR (SR–comparative tissue measurement). The value of the deformation factor means compression. The maximum value of compression in human tissue is 2%. The SR value, or comparative tissue measurement, indicates how much the tissue in the test area is harder or softer than the tissue in the reference test area. From these values, the means were calculated and used for statistical calculations (Figure 1).

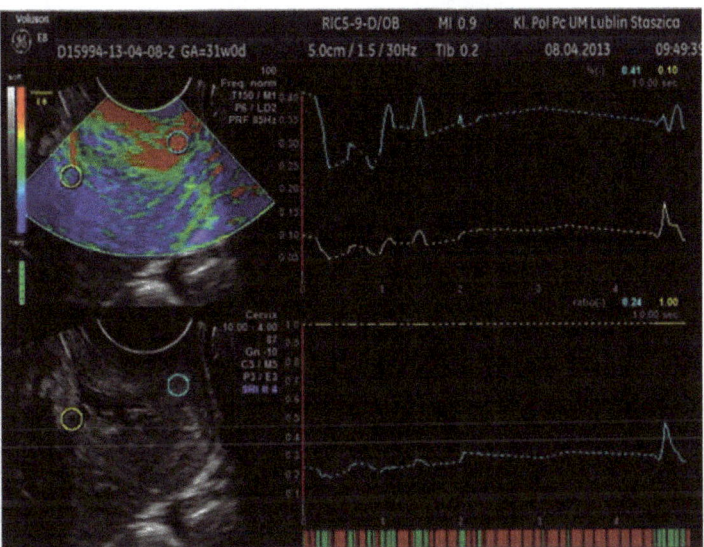

Figure 1. Cervical elastographic evaluation in the Elastography Analysis program.

The transducer receives two sets of radiofrequency signals: before and after squeezing the cervix, and the amount of shift in the tissue is estimated from the waveform difference. Tissue rate versus distance from the transducer is calculated for all image points. The rate of change values are known as strain values and are displayed in a variety of colors ranging from red to yellow, green to blue for soft and hard tissues. Tissues marked in red are considered to be the most flexible tissues, while tissues with the least elasticity are marked in blue (Figure 2).

Laboratory tests were performed concurrently with the ultrasound examinations. These studies used serum samples separated from peripheral blood and samples of cervical secretions obtained from the simultaneous collection from a given patient.

Blood from the antecubital vein was collected in a volume of 9 mL into disposable S-Monovettes (Sarstedt, Germany) containing a blood clotting activator. The solidification process took place at room temperature and lasted approximately 30–40 min. The samples were then centrifuged in a centrifuge (Sigma 1-6P, Polygen) for 10 min at room temperature and 3800 rpm. The serum obtained in this way was aliquoted 200 µL in Eppendorf tubes (Medlab Products) and stored at −75 °C (Platinum Angelantoni 500, Italy) until the measurements were made.

Cervical discharge was collected with a sterile swab (Deltalab, Barcelona, Spain) while examined in a sterile speculum from the posterior vaginal fornix. If vaginal discharge could not be collected, a sample was collected from the cervix. A swab was inserted into the outer mouth of the cervix to a depth of 1–2 cm and then pressing the mucous membrane several times (for 10–15 s), which allowed for the absorption of the appropriate amount of secretion. The material collected in this way was placed in a sterile, tightly closed tube and sent to a laboratory.

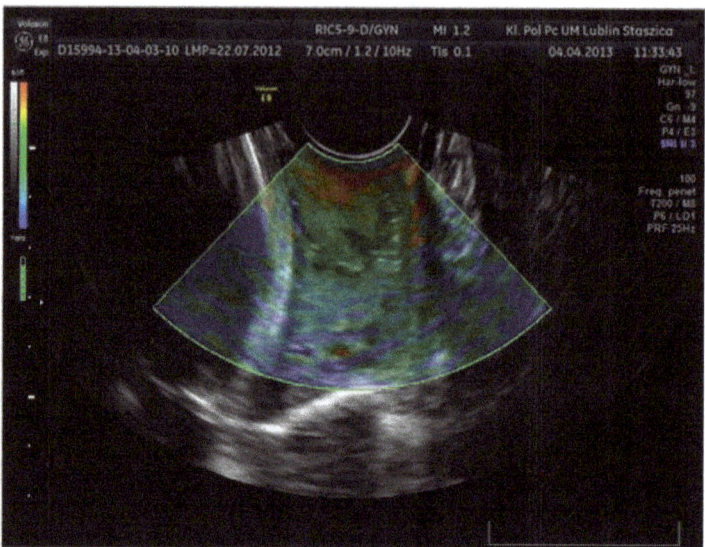

Figure 2. Cervical elastographic assessment. Tissue elasticity distribution calculations in real-time and presented using a color scale—red (soft), blue (hard), and green (medium-hard).

In the next step, the swab with the sample was transferred to a tube containing 2 mL of PBS (Phosphate Buffered Saline (PAA Laboratories GmbH, Leonding, Austria) without calcium (Ca^{2+}) and magnesium (Mg^{2+}) ions). The secretion was extracted by vigorously rotating the swab inside the tube for about 10 s, and then the samples were centrifuged for 10 min at room temperature, at a speed of 3800 rpm. The supernatant thus obtained was collected from the sediment and aliquoted 200 µL. The material was stored in the same way as in the case of the serum.

Determination of the concentration of metalloproteinases 8 (MMP-8) and 9 (MMP-9) in the tested material was performed with the use of commercially available ELISA kits (Enzyme-linked Immunosorbent Assay) based on immunological reactions. All test steps were performed in accordance with the procedures recommended by the manufacturer of the assay kits. The following test was used to determine the concentration of MMP-8: Quantikine Human Total MMP-8 Immunoassay. For the quantitative determination of human active and pro-Matrix Metalloproteinase 8 (total MMP-8) concentrations in cell culture supernatants, serum, plasma, and saliva, Cat # DMP800 was used (R&D Systems Europe Ltd., Abingdon, UK). The mean analytical sensitivity of the assay was 0.02 ng/mL (0.01 to 0.06 ng/mL), and the measuring range was from 0 to 10 ng/mL (lowest concentration to highest standard concentration).

The following assay was used to determine the level of MMP-9: Quantikine Human MMP-9 Immunoassay. For the quantitative determination of human active (82 kDa) and Pro- (92 kDa) Matrix Metalloproteinase 9 (MMP-9) concentrations in cell culture supernatants, serum, plasma, saliva, and urine, Cat # DMP900 was used (R&D Systems Europe Ltd., Abingdon, UK).

The sensitivity of the assay, defined as the minimum detectable dose (MDD) of human MMP-9, was less than 0.156 ng/mL. The measuring range was from 0 to 20 ng/mL (from the lowest concentration to the highest standard concentration).

A statistical analysis of clinical data was performed using: the arithmetic mean standard deviation (SD), medians (ME) using the Shapiro–Wilk test, and the Kruskal-Wallis H test. A comparison of the differences between the control group and the study group was carried out with the Student's *t*-test. For the variables tested, which did not show normal distribution, non-parametric tests were used for further analysis. The concentrations of

MMP-8 and MMP-9 were compared using the U-Mann-Whitney test and the Pearson Chi2 test. The relationship between individual substances and clinical data was carried out using the Spearman correlation test. Statistical significance was set at $p \leq 0.05$. Results statistically insignificant were defined by the abbreviation "ns". Statistical calculations were based on Statistica 10 (StatSoft, Tulsa, OK, USA).

4. Results

Characteristics of the Study and Control Groups

The study group included 58 pregnant women at risk of preterm labor, while the control group included 30 healthy pregnant women with a physiological course of pregnancy. Based on medical records, questionnaires, and an interview, demographic, social, and clinical data were collected for each patient participating in the study. The demographic, socio-clinical characteristics of the study and control groups are presented in Tables 1–3.

Table 1. Demographic, socio-clinical characteristics of the study and control group.

Parameter		Study No (n)	Control No (n)	Study Percentage (%)	Control Percentage (%)
Age	20–30 yo	38	19	63..33	66.67
	31–40 yo	19	11	36.67	33.33
Education	Secondary	10	1	3.33	17.54
	Higher	47	6	20	82.46
Place of living	Rural	18	23	76.67	31.58
	Urban < 100,000 people	14	11	36.67	24.56
	Urban > 100,000 people	25	6	20	43.86
Employment	Employed	28	13	43.33	49.12
	Unemployed	29	16	53.33	5.88
Number of pregnancies	1	37	14	46.67	64.91
	2	14	16	53.33	24.56
	3	4	9	30	7.02
	4	2	3	10	3.51
Number of deliveries	1	41	2	6.67	71.93
	2	15	17	56.67	26.32
	3	1	11	36.67	1.75
High-risk factors	N/A	29	2	6.67	50.88
	PTB in family	7	18	60	12.28
	Infertility	6	1	3.33	10.53
	Miscarriage	6	3	10	10.53
	PTB	3	1	3.33	5.26
	Cervical incompetence	3	2	6.67	5.26
	Urinary and vaginal tract infection	3	2	6.67	5.26
	FGR		1		3.33
	Hypothyroidism		1		3.33
	Uterine myomas		1		3.33

Abbreviations: yo—year old, N/A—not applicable, PTB—preterm birth, FGR—Fetal Growth Restriction.

Table 2. Detailed characteristics of the study group in terms of selected demographic and clinical parameters.

Parameter	N	Average	Median	Min	Max	SD
Age (years) *	57	29.70	30	22	39	3.93
Duration of gestation (wks)	57	36.79	38	25	41	4.10
Length of cervix (mm)	57	17.49	19	2	30	6.34
Deformation	57	0.20	0.17	0.01	0.94	0.14
SR-comparative tissue measurement	57	0.83	0.59	0.03	3.86	0.77
MMP-8 serum (ng/mL)	57	74.17	61.63	16.59	287.77	51.50
MMP-8 cervix (ng/mL)	57	155.46	158.34	2.07	379.58	123.14
MMP-9 serum (ng/mL)	57	1308.98	1181.90	418.94	2569.52	591.88
MMP-9 cervix (ng/mL)	57	202.43	103.04	1.72	1258.57	281.85

*—data with a normal distribution (assessed with the Shapiro–Wilk test). N—number of cases, SD—standard deviation

Table 3. Detailed characteristics of the control group in terms of selected demographic and clinical parameters.

Parameter	No	Average	Median	Min	Max	SD
Age (years) *	27	30.74	30	25	39	4.07
Duration of gestation (wks)	30	39.10	40	28	41	2.26
Length of cervix * (mm)	30	34.73	34	25	46	6.37
Deformation	30	0.20	0.16	0.009	0.61	0.13
SR—comparative tissue measurement	30	1.23	0.57	0.17	6.56	1.65
MMP-8 serum (ng/mL) *	30	58.44	57.47	14.99	123.73	26.22
MMP-8 cervix (ng/mL)	30	94.19	60.95	1.14	259.02	91.08
MMP-9 serum (ng/mL) *	30	1261.56	1134.42	447.30	2258.83	505.83
MMP-9 cervix(ng/mL)	30	103.59	59.70	2.24	554.40	122.21

*—data with a normal distribution (assessed with the Shapiro–Wilk test). WKS—weeks gestation

The comparison of the distribution of values of selected demographic and clinical parameters in the study and control groups showed statistically significant differences in the variables—duration of pregnancy, CL, and MMP-8 concentration (assessed in samples of cervical secretion collected from the posterior vaginal fornix). It was noted that the parameter duration of pregnancy in weeks had significantly higher values in the control group than in the study group (40 (95% CI: 39–40) vs. 38 (95% CI: 37–39) weeks; test value U = 451 0; test value Z = −3.6; significance level p = 0.0002). Figure 3 shows a comparison of the parameter value the duration of pregnancy in weeks in the study and control groups. Similarly, the variable CL in mm had significantly higher values in the control group compared to the study group (34 (95% CI: 30, 17–39) vs. 19 (95% CI: 16–21) mm; test value U = 12.0; test value Z = −7.52; significance level p < 0.0001). In the case of the other examined variables, no statistically significant differences were found in the distribution of data. A graph comparing the value of the variable neck length in the test and control groups is presented in Figure 4.

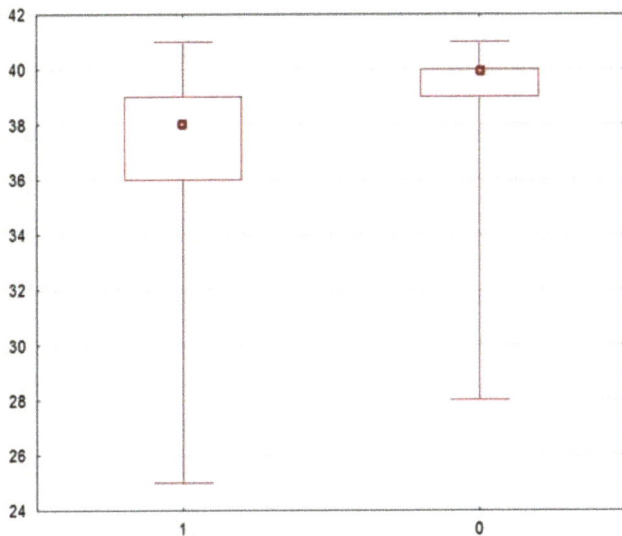

Figure 3. A box-whisker chart showing the comparison of the duration of pregnancy (wks) parameter in the study-1 and control-0 groups.

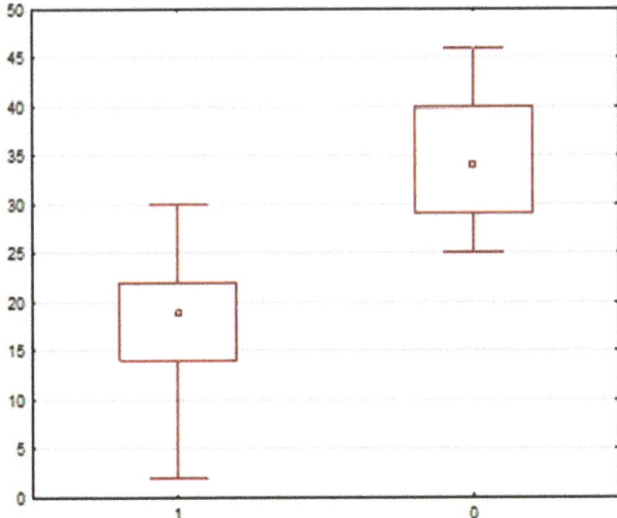

Figure 4. A box-whisker chart showing a comparison of the value of the variable cervical length—mm in the study-1 and control-0 groups.

However, in the case of MMP-8 concentration significantly lower values of this parameter were observed in the control group compared to the study group (60.95 (95% CI: 25.38–89.86) vs. 158.34 (95% CI: 61.81–216.99) ng/mL; U test value = 631.5 Z test value = 1.99 and significance level p = 0.0459. Presented in Figure 5.

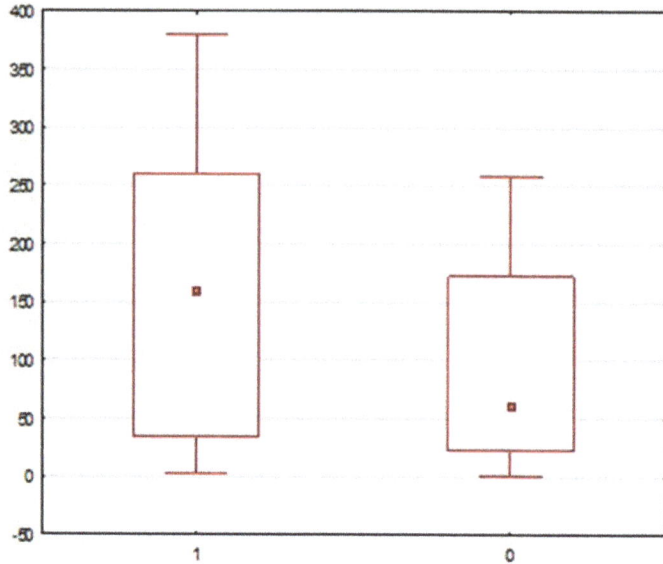

Figure 5. A box-whisker plot showing a comparison of MMP-8 ng/mL concentrations (assessed in cervical samples) in the study-1 and control-0 groups.

Based on the data analysis, several correlations were observed between the selected demographic and clinical parameters in the study group. There was a statistically significant mean negative correlation between the strain values and the SR-comparative tissue measurement (rho = −0.4248; p = 0.0010). Moreover, a statistically significant, average positive correlation was observed between the values of the cervix length and the parameter of pregnancy duration (wks) (rho = 0.3729; p = 0.0043). A very high positive correlation was also found between the concentration of MMP-8, and MMP-9 assessed in the peripheral blood serum (rho = 0.8387; p < 0.0001). A very high positive correlation was also observed in the case of MMP-8 and MMP-9 concentrations assessed in samples of cervical secretion from the posterior vaginal fornix (rho = 0.7798; p < 0.001). In the case of the remaining possible combinations of MMP-8 MMP-9 concentrations in peripheral blood serum and samples taken from the cervix, no statistically significant correlations were found. On the other hand, there were several correlations between demographic and clinical variables and the concentrations of MMP-8 and MMP-9 assessed in various study materials and an average negative correlation between MMP-8 values assessed in the cervical material and the age of the examined patients (rho = −0.4000; p = 0.0020). The age of the respondents also negatively correlated with the values of MMP-9 concentrations assessed in the material taken from the cervix (however, it was a weak correlation) (rho = −0.2986; p = 0.02). Similarly, a weak negative correlation was observed between the values of the parameters of the duration of pregnancy and MMP-9 (assessed in the material taken from the posterior vaginal vault) (rho = −0.3434; p = 0.0089).

Based on the data analysis, several correlations were observed between the selected demographic and clinical parameters in the control group. There was a statistically significant negative correlation between the values of SR parameters, comparative measurement of tissues, and cervical length (rho = −0.3743; p = 0.0416).

As in the study group, a high positive correlation was found between the concentration of MMP-8 and MMP-9 assessed in the peripheral blood serum (rho = 0.7511; p < 0.0001). A high positive correlation was also observed in the case of MMP-8 and MMP-9 concentrations assessed in samples of cervical secretion from the posterior vaginal fornix (rho = 0.5189; p = 0.0033). No statistically significant correlations were found for the remaining possible combinations of MMP-8 and MMP-9 concentrations in peripheral blood serum and samples taken from the posterior vaginal fornix.

There were, however, two correlations between clinical variables and the values of MMP-8 concentrations assessed in samples taken from the cervix.

Among other things, there was an average negative correlation between the MMP-8 values assessed in the cervical material and the SR parameter—comparative tissue measurement in the control group (rho = −0.3737; p = 0.0419). There was also an average negative correlation between MMP-8 values assessed in the material collected from the posterior vaginal fornix and the parameter—duration of pregnancy in weeks (rho = 0.3623; p = 0.0491). Based on the analysis carried out with the use of ROC curves, it was found that among the studied demographic and clinical variables, only the length of the cervix (in mm) and the concentration of MMP-8 (in ng/mL), assessed in the cervical secretion obtained from the posterior vaginal fornix, were significantly high in the area under the curve (AUC) value in the early detection of the possibility of preterm labor.

For the cut-off value of the cervical parameter length $\leq$ 26 mm determined on the basis of the ROC curve, the sensitivity and specificity of the detection of preterm labor were 98.2% and 96.7%, respectively (AUC = 0.993, 95% CI: 0.437–0.659; p < 0.0001; Figure 6). On the other hand, in the case of the cut-off value for MMP-8 concentration assessed in peripheral blood serum > 90.8 ng/mL, the sensitivity and specificity of preterm labor detection were 57.9% and 70%, respectively (AUC = 0.631, 95% CI: 0.520–0.732; p < 0.0291; Figure 7). On the other hand, the other examined variables (sensitivity and specificity, respectively): age (94.7% and 18.5%), strain (84.2% and 23.3%), SR—comparative tissue measurement (38.6% and 63, 3%), concentrations of MMP-8 (33.3% and 86.7%) and MMP-9 (47.4% and 66.7%) assessed in peripheral blood serum, and the concentration of MMP-9 (21.1% and 96.7%), tested in samples from the cervix, proved to be insignificantly diagnostic in detecting preterm labor (Figures 6–13). Detailed data on the assessment of the diagnostic usefulness of selected demographic and clinical factors using ROC curves are presented in Table 4.

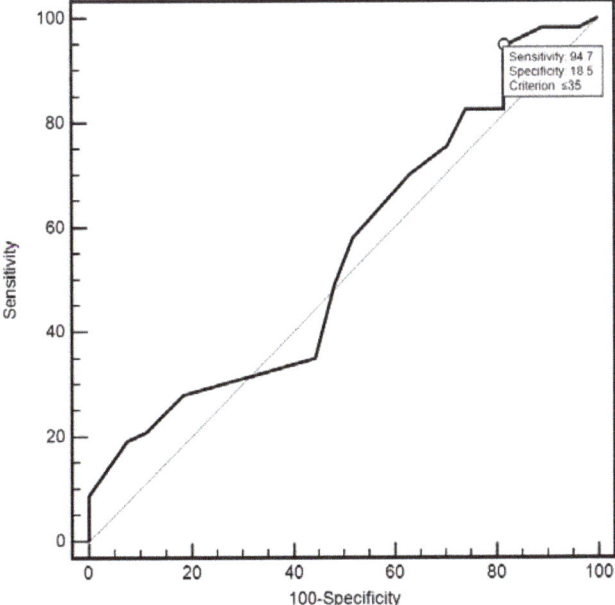

Figure 6. Diagnostic usefulness of the age parameter in the early detection of preterm labor using the ROC curve.

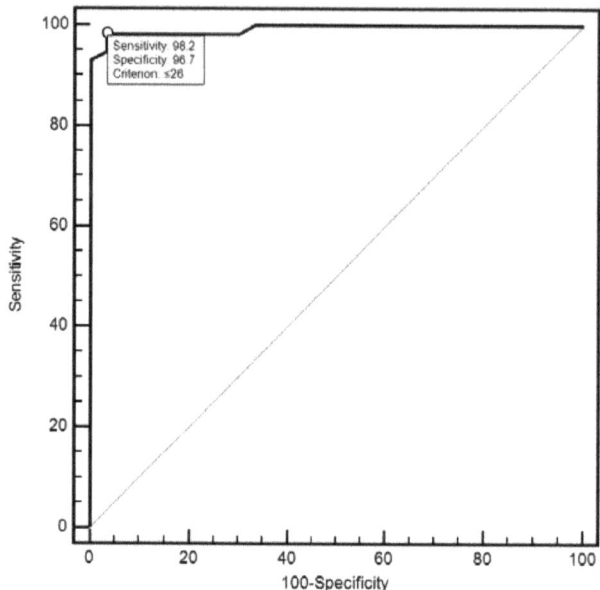

Figure 7. Assessment of the diagnostic usefulness of the cervical length parameter in early detection of preterm labor using the ROC curve.

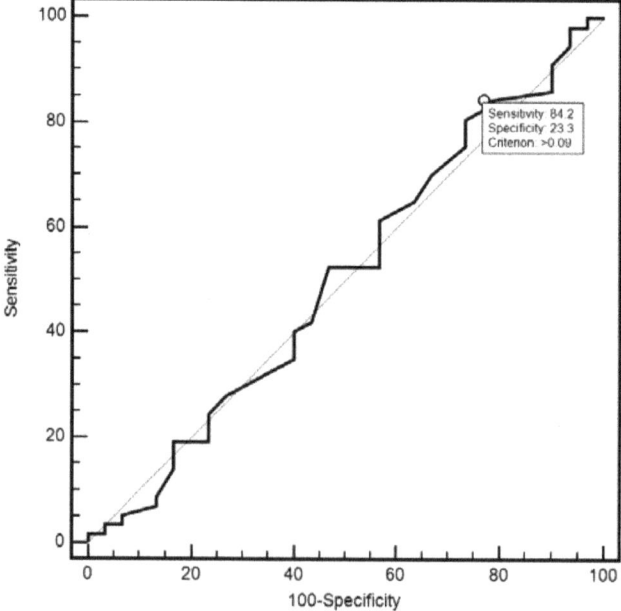

Figure 8. Evaluation of the diagnostic usefulness of the deformity parameter in the early detection of preterm labor using the ROC curve.

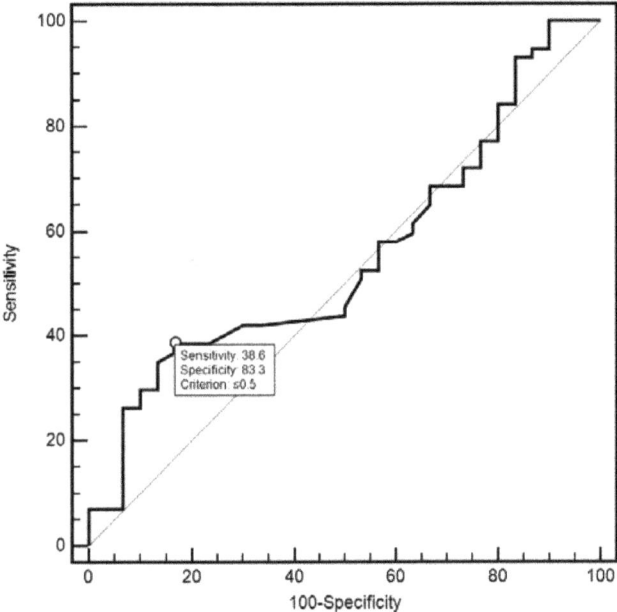

Figure 9. Diagnostic usefulness of the SR parameter—comparative tissue measurement in the early detection of preterm labor using the ROC curve.

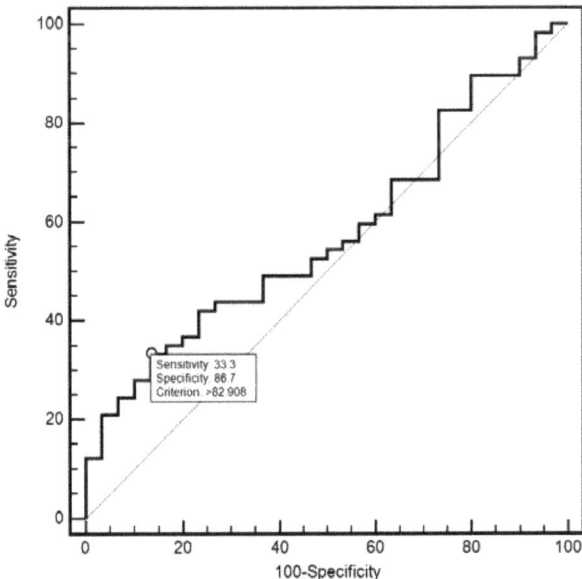

Figure 10. Assessment of the diagnostic usefulness of the MMP-8 (ng/mL) concentration determination in the peripheral blood serum in the early detection of preterm labor using the ROC curve.

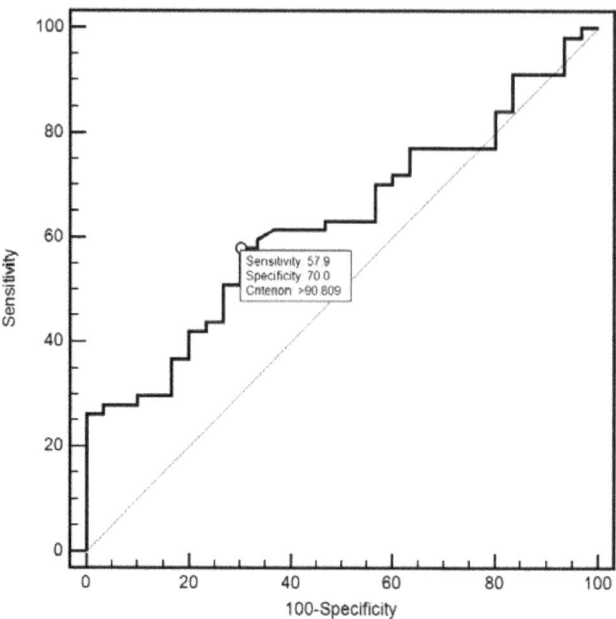

Figure 11. Evaluation of the diagnostic usefulness of MMP-8 (ng/mL) concentration determination in samples taken from the cervix in early detection of preterm labor using the ROC curve.

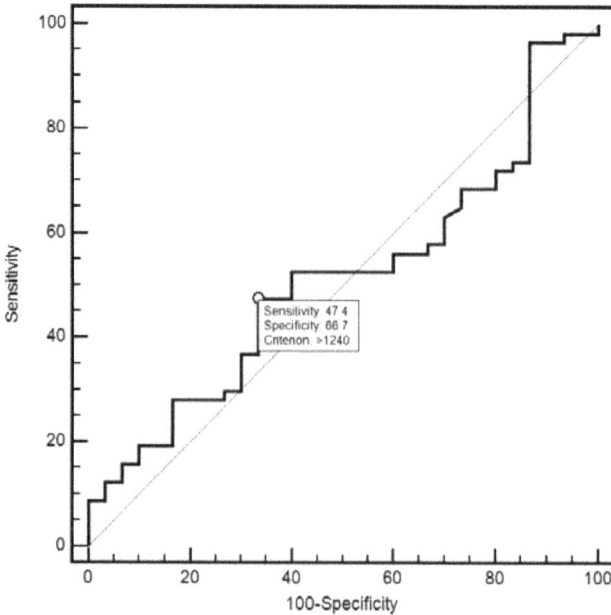

Figure 12. Assessment of the diagnostic usefulness of the MMP-9 (ng/mL) concentration determination in the peripheral blood serum in the early detection of preterm labor using the ROC curve.

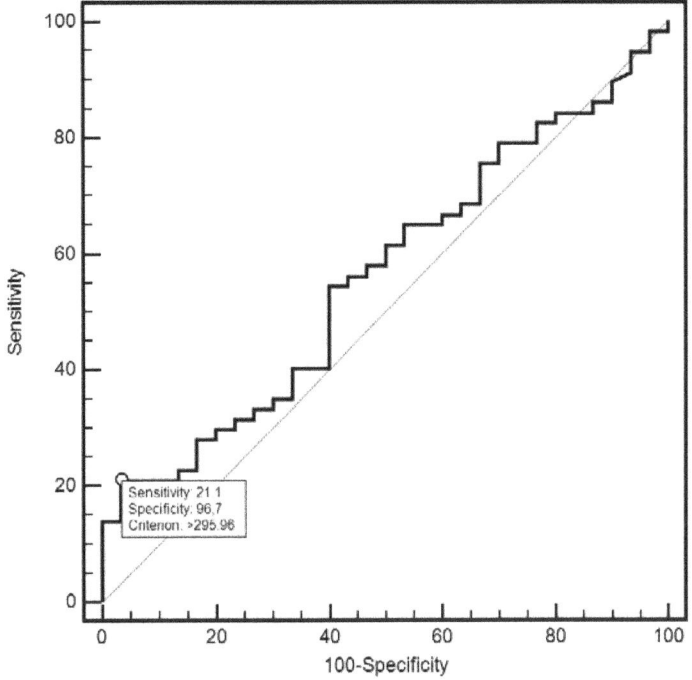

Figure 13. Evaluation of the diagnostic usefulness of MMP-9 (ng/mL) concentration determination in samples taken from the cervix in the early detection of preterm labor using the ROC curve.

Table 4. Characteristics of the parameters of ROC curves for the concentration values of MMP-8 cervical (ng/mL).

Parameter	AUC	SE	95%CI	Level (AUC = 0.5)
Age (years)	0.550	0.068	0.437–0.659	0.4674
Cervical length (mm)	0.993	0.006	0.945–1.000	<0.0001
Deformation	0.506	0.067	0.397–0.615	0.9240
SR-comparative tissue measurement	0.553	0.064	0.443–0.660	0.4067
MMP-8 cervix (ng/mL)	0.631	0.059	0.520–0.732	0.0291
MMP-8 serum (ng/mL)	0.575	0.062	0.465–0.681	0.2275
MMP-9 cervix (ng/mL)	0.562	0.063	0.452–0.668	0.3266
MMP-9 serum (ng/mL)	0.514	0.064	0.405–0.623	0.8236

AUC—Area Under the Curve, SE—standard error, CI—confidence interval.

5. Discussion

Despite a significant development that has taken place in recent years in medicine, preterm labor still remains one of the major problems of modern obstetrics and therefore is one of the most serious challenges of modern perinatology (1). The aim of this study was to assess the effects of biochemical markers and ultrasound measurement on predicting preterm labor. The physical markers included the assessment of cervical length and its elastographic assessment, while the biochemical factors included the assessment of the concentration of metalloproteinases in the vaginal-cervical secretion and in the maternal blood serum. Statistical analysis of the age of the patients did not show statistically significant differences. The test and control groups were homogeneous in terms of age.

In the study group, the mean age was 29.7 years. However, in the control group, the mean age was slightly higher, amounting to 30.7 years). The age of the patients had no significant effect on the increased risk of preterm labor. Most of the scientific reports, analyzing the data on patients with extreme age, confirm the fact that the age of the patients influences the risk of preterm labor [26,27]. In a study by Cooper et al., obstetric results were assessed in very young 15-year-old married women with secondary education, white race, under medical care [26]. Similarly, Astolfi et al. Comparing the age of parents at 20–29 years with the age of the mother over 30 and the father over 40 showed that the influence of paternal age on the risk of preterm labor is smaller but significant if he is over 40 [28]. It is noteworthy that the deformation parameter (cervical) was slightly higher in older patients, but this relationship did not become statistically significant.

In this research, the variable "duration of pregnancy" in the study and control group was compared with the variable "cervical length" assessed in the ultrasound examination. It was confirmed that the parameter "duration of pregnancy in weeks" had significantly higher values in the control group compared to the study group. It was shown that in patients whose variable "cervical length" was less than or equal to 25 mm, the parameter "duration of pregnancy" in weeks had statistically significantly lower values. The obtained results lead to the conclusion that the CL expressed in millimeters is inversely proportional to the risk of preterm labor. This is confirmed by the Berghella study, according to which screening the length of the cervix with transvaginal ultrasound is a good prognostic test for the prediction of spontaneous preterm labor in single pregnancies with symptoms of preterm labor [29]. It has been shown that in patients at risk of preterm labor, for whom the cervical length measurement is known, the incidence of spontaneous preterm labor is lower, and the gestational age at delivery is higher. This is due to the possibility of using appropriate clinical management. Asymptomatic women at risk should be screened at a 2-week interval starting from 16 to 18 weeks, up to 24 weeks. CLs < 10th centile are at risk of PTB, especially with a decrease in CL after 16 weeks [30]

In our study, the results of the ultrasound assessment of the CL and an elastographic examination were analyzed. The evaluation of the cervical length measurement in relation to other parameters is the subject of many studies comparing the palpation with ultrasound examination of the cervix, especially in patients with premature contractions of the uterine muscle and preserved amniotic fluid [31–34]. Women between 24 and 34 weeks of pregnancy were assessed. On admission to the hospital, the cervix was assessed in relation to the Bishop scale and the length of the cervix measured by ultrasound in all patients. Statistical analysis showed a difference based on cervical evaluation methods. More medical information was provided by the results of ultrasound examinations. However, both methods had a similar predictive value [32]. In our study, the cervix was not assessed according to the Bishop score due to the subjectivity of this method, emphasized by other authors [33,34]. Similar results were obtained in the Pedretti screening [35]. It assessed the length of the cervix in ultrasound in asymptomatic patients. It has been confirmed that this form of examination can be successfully used to identify asymptomatic patients with single pregnancies at risk of preterm labor.

The aim of this study was to confirm the hypothesis of the existence of a correlation between the so-called "Soft cervix" in the elastographic evaluation and its reduced length, and therefore the use of elastography as a marker of premature labor. One of the inspirations for this assumption was a study conducted by Thomas et al. in 2007 in non-pregnant women, who assessed the elasticity of neoplastic changes in the cervix and, for the first time, used the elastographic technique to assess the cervix [36]. Thomas et al. created a cervical pattern. Measurements were made with a transvaginal probe with slight compression of the cervix. The elastographic images were analyzed using a program that allows semi-quantitative tissue stiffness analysis. Tissue elasticity distribution calculations were performed in real-time and presented using a color scale—red (soft), blue (hard), and green (medium-hard). Based on this study, it was determined that cervical neoplastic changes can be identified as less flexible structures within the cervix. The hypothesis of our research was based on the assumption that there is a dependence of cervical elasticity on the extent of pregnancy. Unfortunately, the evaluation of the correlation of parameters such as strain and SR, i.e., a comparative measurement of the tissues determining the consistency of the cervix with the "duration of pregnancy", proved to be statistically insignificant. Therefore, the above-mentioned parameters are not good markers of preterm labor. The results on the basis of which this conclusion was drawn were calculated based on the analysis performed with the use of ROC curves. Similar research results were obtained by Maurer et al., who showed a very weak correlation between elastography and clinical features of the population, such as a history of preterm labor and cervical length less than 30 mm [37]. Due to the non-standardized values of the force exerted by the probe on the cervix, only an assessment of the relative formability within each organ can be obtained. Therefore, this study does not provide information about the evolution of changes in the elasticity of the entire organ because it does not lead to the normalization of the strength as the color scale signal depends on the imaged deformation, i.e., the susceptibility of the examined tissues. Based on the tests performed with the Voluson E8 apparatus, using the RIC5-9-D endovaginal probe with static elastography software, it was impossible to obtain the same tissue deformation forces during one ultrasound examination with the use of elastography, which conditioned the obtaining of comparable results, even when examined by the same person. Therefore, in the case of the calculated coefficients, mean values were taken into account, which were included in the statistical calculations. Fruscalzo et al. proposed standardization of the ROI area and developed guidelines for controlling the effect of a force applied with a transvaginal probe [38,39]. The ROI was placed across the entire thickness of the cervical anterior lip to reduce the variation due to tissue heterogeneity and force dispersion due to the distance from the transvaginal probe. Thus, it was possible to quantify cervical deformity on a continuous scale of values. In turn, Parra-Saavedra et al. calculated the cervical consistency index (CCI). In his study, he used the anteroposterior thickness of the cervix (AP), measured before and after applying pressure to the cervix, respectively [40]. A significant relationship between CCI and the elastographic assessment of the cervix was also confirmed in the study by Mazza et al. [34]. The above-mentioned authors emphasize that the deformation coefficient depends on the distance between the ROI frame and the transvaginal probe, i.e., the greater the elasticity of the test center, the less repeatable the test is. Therefore, in our study, the reference point of reference was the hard parts of the fetus (skull bones), considering them as reference areas in relation to the cervix due to similar bone mineralization in a given week of pregnancy. The results of our own research showed an identical deformation coefficient for both groups. On the other hand, SR, i.e., the comparative tissue measurement, differed slightly between the studied groups but did not reach the level of statistical significance. The obtained results did not show a relationship between tissue elasticity and the duration of pregnancy and did not confirm the hypothesis that the less elastic the cervical tissue, the lower the risk of preterm labor.

Promising research, opposed to our own research, was Nicolaides's group's 2012 analysis. Its purpose was to confirm the objectivity of the elastographic examination. The repeatability of elastographic measurements was then assessed. Two investigators assessed the cervixes of the same pregnant women. No statistically significant differences were found in the elastographic measurements by both researchers, except for the area that directly perceived the power of the transducer. On the basis of the conducted analysis, it was concluded that an objective assessment of the cervical elastogram is possible [33]. It seems, however, that the elastographic evaluation of the neck has some limitations, as the studies conducted by the author did not confirm the conclusions resulting from the above-mentioned analyzes. No statistically significant correlation was found between the value of the parameters assessed and the length of the cervix and the duration of pregnancy; therefore, the usefulness of elastography in a clinical study in predicting preterm labor was not demonstrated. Moreover, in the study group, a negative correlation between the values of deformation and the SR measurement of tissues was noted, and in the control group, a negative correlation between the values of SR parameters—comparative measurement of tissues and the length of the cervix. This did not allow for a clear comparison of the two groups in terms of the above-mentioned correlations and thus to draw conclusions about the usefulness of this study in predicting preterm labor.

Further studies are needed to evaluate the suitability of this technique for clinical application, such as predicting preterm labor or successful induction of labor. In our own study, the elastographic evaluation used a numerical scale obtained in the Elastography Analysis program. However, elastographic maps in terms of color were not assessed, as was done, for instance by Woźniak et al. [41]. The above-mentioned researchers found that elastographic evaluation of the internal cervix in 18–22 weeks of pregnancy in patients with shortened cervix may be useful in predicting premature labor. The hardness of the inner orifice of the cervix was assessed elastographically using a color scale: red (soft), yellow (medium-soft), blue (medium-hard), and purple (hard). In the case of visualization of two colors around the inner mouth, the softer option was chosen. The following variables were analyzed: the percentage of premature births in the different categories of internal orifice hardness and the sensitivity, specificity, negative and positive predictive value of elastography in predicting preterm labor. The number of premature deliveries was significantly higher in the red group than in the blue and purple groups. The cut-off point for elastography suggests adopting both red and yellow colors as factors predisposing to preterm labor. The comparison of both methods (elastographic map and numerical scale) is not really possible. The parameters assessed in the own study (deformation and SR—comparative tissue measurement) in the study group showed a statistically significant average negative correlation with each other, which does not allow for drawing unequivocal conclusions. No results were obtained that would confirm the conclusions formulated by the authors. However, it should be taken into account that the methods used by the author differed radically from the methods used by Woźniak et al., as can be seen, elastography seems to be a promising diagnostic method.

Unfortunately, there is still no consensus on the optimal method for assessing the cervix. Virtually most of the previous studies, evaluating the use of various elastography methods, gave many satisfactory results [42–44].

In this study, the relationship between the concentration of metalloproteinases in blood serum and vaginal-cervical secretions in pregnant women was analyzed. Most studies analyze the concentration of MMP-8 and MMP-9 in the amniotic fluid in association with other fluid components and their correlation with preterm labor. The latest one aimed at investigating the association of MMP-1, MMP-8 and MMP-9 polymorphisms, and levels of MMP-9 in preterm birth with positive results [45]. A study by Lee et al. found that a model combining the concentration of various amniotic fluid proteins, including MMP-8 and MMP-9, with clinical factors can improve the accuracy of preterm labor prediction [46]. Moreover, the assessment of these correlations is more accurate than the assessment of single biomarkers in women with cervical insufficiency. The concentration of MMP-8 in the cervical secretion was significantly higher in the study group as compared to the control group. Therefore, it can be concluded that the measurement of MMP-8 concentration can be one of the methods of predicting preterm labor, as was stated in research by Lee and Park [47]. Yoo et al. also assessed the concentration of metalloproteinases in the cervicovaginal secretion. He showed that proteins involved in immune regulation, including MMP-8 and MMP-9, alone or in combination with clinical risk factors, may be useful as predictors of spontaneous preterm labor in women with cervical insufficiency or with an ultrasound short cervix (≤ 25 mm) [48]. The combination of these markers and clinical factors significantly improves the predictability of preterm labor compared to the markers alone. The results obtained in our own study confirm the above-mentioned concept. A statistically significant positive correlation was found between the cervical length values and the duration of pregnancy, and it was also confirmed that the concentration of MMP-8 in the uterine cervical discharge is significantly higher in the study group compared to the control group. Therefore, it can be concluded that measuring the concentration of MMP-8 together with the evaluation of the cervix may be useful markers of preterm labor.

Scientific studies have shown that in pregnancy, the concentration of matrix metalloproteinases in the cervical mucus is statistically higher [49]. However, their physiological and pathophysiological significance is not fully understood and elucidated, although it has been proven that the concentrations of MMP-8 and MMP-9 increase mainly in the distal part of the mucous plug depending on the stages of pregnancy. It seems that it is related to the defense against infectious agents acting mainly in this area of the cervix. In patients delivering prematurely, the concentrations of MMP-8, MMP-9, and IL-8 in the cervical secretion are several times higher compared to the concentrations of these substances in the mucous plugs of patients delivering at term. As there are different molecular mechanisms underlying preterm labor without and from damage to the membranes, the concentration of MMP-8 in the cervical secretion may thus reflect the different functions of this protease. Therefore, the use of MMP-8 to differentiate the causes of preterm labor is not recommended [50]. However, it does not change the fact that MMP-8 can be effectively used as a marker of premature labor.

In our study, the group of patients was quite heterogeneous in terms of the cause of preterm labor, and yet in all patients, the concentration of this metalloproteinase was significantly increased in the cervical secretion. On the other hand, the concentration of metalloproteinases in the peripheral blood serum of this dissertation is consistent with the results obtained by other researchers and does not show significant differences between patients with a physiological pregnancy and patients with a risk of premature delivery [51]. In this study, the concentrations of MMP-9 in the blood serum and in the cervical secretion were assessed. It would seem that the concentrations of MMP-9 should statistically significantly differ between the study group and the control group. Unfortunately, the tested material did not provide any results confirming this thesis. The concentration of MMP-9 in the blood serum in patients in the study group did not differ significantly from the concentration of MMP-9 in the control group, although the difference between the concentration in the cervical secretion collected from the posterior vaginal fornix in the study group was slightly higher, but not statistically significant. Athayde et al. conducted a study to determine whether the increased bioavailability of MMP-9 was associated with preterm labor [52]. The results were as follows: spontaneous delivery at term was associated with a statistically significant increase, and the concentration of MMP-9 in the amniotic fluid was statistically higher in the group of women with preterm labor compared to the group of women with the risk of preterm delivery, who gave birth at the expected date of delivery. Moreover, MMP-9 concentrations did not change with the progressive gestational age. In conclusion, a significant increase in MMP-9 concentration is characteristic of PPROM (preterm premature rupture of membranes); therefore, MMP-9 cannot be considered a marker of preterm labor. This concept is also confirmed by the results of our study. The study conducted by the authors showed differences in the concentrations of both metalloproteinases in the study group as compared to the control group; however, both groups were not analyzed in terms of the etiopathogenetic factor of preterm labor, i.e., infection. The concentrations of MMP-8 and MMP-9 in the cervical secretion were higher in patients in the study group; the concentrations of MMP-8 were significantly higher while the concentrations of MMP-9 differed slightly. Similar results were obtained by Myntti et al., but in his study, the cause of preterm labor was important [53]. This study assessed the proteolytic biomarkers of the amniotic fluid that form the inflammatory cascade in response to microbial invasion of the amniotic cavity and intrauterine infection in preterm labor with intact membranes. The research results obtained by the author indicate that the concentrations of MMP-8, MMP-9 (and others) were higher in the case of suspected infection compared to the control group and also in the case of intrauterine infection. The tested biomarkers, including MMP-8 and MMP-9, had a sensitivity of 100% with thresholds based on the ROC curve. The analysis of the study group indicates that in some patients, the cause of preterm labor could be an intrauterine infection.

Metalloproteinases are involved in the pathogenesis of preterm labor but are not only related to intrauterine birth. Therefore, an increase in their concentrations may be an important predictive factor, especially in the case of MMP-8 not related to the infectious nature of preterm labor. The results of the authors' research indicate that the monitoring of the length of the cervix and the non-invasive assessment of biochemical markers of preterm labor, including metalloproteinases, may allow for the personalization of pregnancies at risk of preterm labor and, in the long term, also enable effective prevention of a number of serious perinatal complications. Delivery and proper postnatal care in properly equipped perinatal centers, as well as timely implemented therapeutic interventions, can significantly reduce the incidence of preterm labor and the effects of prematurity.

6. Conclusions

Assessment of the cervical length plays a key role in the ultrasound assessment of cervical length and is one of the most important markers of preterm labor. The use of static elastography does not meet the criterion of a good marker of premature labor in high-risk patients. However, in the same group of patients, the MMP-8 concentration may be one of the methods of predicting preterm labor.

Author Contributions: Conceptualization, I.D.-D., A.K. (Arkadiusz Krzyżanowski) and A.K. (Aleksandra Stupak); methodology, I.D.-D., A.K. (Aleksandra Stupak) and A.K. (Arkadiusz Krzyżanowski); software, T.G.; validation, I.D.-D., and A.S.; formal analysis, A.S.; investigation, I.D.-D., A.K. (Adrianna Kondracka), T.G. and A.S.; resources, T.G., and A.K. (Anna Kwaśniewska); data curation, I.D.-D., A.K. (Adrianna Kondracka), T.G. and A.S.; writing—original draft preparation, I.D.-D. and A.S.; writing—review and editing, A.K. (Arkadiusz Krzyżanowski) and A.K. (Anna Kwaśniewska); visualization, A.S. and T.G.; supervision, A.K. (Arkadiusz Krzyżanowski) and A.K. (Anna Kwaśniewska); project administration, A.K. (Anna Kwaśniewska); funding acquisition, A.K. (Anna Kwaśniewska). All authors have read and agreed to the published version of the manuscript.

Funding: This work was supported by the Medical University of Lublin, Poland, under Grant DS 120.

Institutional Review Board Statement: The study was conducted according to the guidelines of the Declaration of Helsinki, and approved by the Ethics Committee of Medical University of Lublin, Poland (KE-0254/134/2009 and KE-0254/294/2017).

Informed Consent Statement: Informed consent was obtained from all subjects involved in the study.

Conflicts of Interest: The authors declare no conflict of interest.

References

1. Walani, S.R. Global burden of preterm birth. *Int. J. Gynecol. Obstet.* **2020**, *150*, 31–33. [CrossRef] [PubMed]
2. Costeloe, K.; EPICure Study Group. EPICure: Facts and figures: Why preterm labour should be treated. *BJOG* **2006**, *113*, 10–12. [CrossRef] [PubMed]
3. The Fetal Medicine Foundation. 2017. Available online: https://fetalmedicine.org/fmf-certification/certificates-of-competence/cervical-assessment-1 (accessed on 27 August 2021).
4. Goldenberg, R.L.; Cliver, S.P.; Mulvihill, F.X.; Hickey, C.A.; Hoffman, H.J.; Klerman, L.V.; Johnson, M.J. Medical, psychosocial, and behavioralrisk factors fpor low birth weight among black woman. *Am. J Obstet. Gynekol.* **1996**, *175*, 1317–1324. [CrossRef]
5. Smith, L.K.; Draper, E.S.; Manktelow, B.N.; Dorling, J.S.; Field, D.J. Socioeconomic inequalities in very preterm birth rates. *Arch. Dis. Child. Fetal Neonatal Ed.* **2007**, *92*, F11–F14. [CrossRef] [PubMed]
6. Hendler, L.; Goldenberg, R.L.; Mercer, B.M.; Iams, J.D.; Meis, P.J.; Moawad, A.H.; MacPherson, C.A.; Caritis, S.N.; Miodovnik, M.; Menard, K.M.; et al. The preterm prediction study: Association between maternal body mass index and spontaneous preterm birth. *Am. J. Obstet. Gynecol.* **2005**, *192*, 882–886. [CrossRef] [PubMed]
7. Goldenberg, R.L.; Culhane, J.F.; Iams, J.D.; Romero, R. Epidemiology and causes of preterm birth. *Lancet* **2008**, *371*, 75–84. [CrossRef]
8. Copper, R.L.; Goldenberg, R.L.; Das, A.; Elder, N.; Swain, M.; Norman, G.; Ramsey, R.; Cotroneo, P.; Collins, B.A.; Johnson, F.; et al. The preterm prediction study: Maternal stress is associated with spontaneous preterm birth at less than thirty five weeks gestation. *Am. J. Obstet. Gynecol.* **1996**, *175*, 1286–1292. [CrossRef]
9. Mozurkewich, E.L.; Luke, B.; Avni, M.; Wolf, F.M. Working conditioned adverse pregnancy outcome: A meta analysis. *Obstret. Gynecol.* **2000**, *95*, 623–625.

10. Krupa, F.G.; Faltin, D.; Cecatti, J.G.; Surita, F.G.C.; Souza, J.P. Predictors of preterm birth. *Int. J. Gynaecol. Obstet.* **2006**, *94*, 5–11. [CrossRef]
11. Saraswat, L.; Ayansina, D.T.; Cooper, K.G.; Bhattacharya, S.; Miligkos, D.; Horne, A.W.; Bhattacharya, S. Pregnancy outcomes in women with endometriosis: A national record linkage study. *BJOG* **2017**, *124*, 444–452. [CrossRef]
12. Romero, R.; Espinoza, J.; Kusanovic, J.P.; Gotsch, F.; Hassan, S.; Erez, O.; Chaiworapongsa, T.; Mazor, M. The preterm parturition syndrome. *BJOG* **2006**, *113*, 17–42. [CrossRef] [PubMed]
13. Kedzierska-Markowicz, A.; Krekora, M.; Biesiada, L.; Głowacka, E.; Krasomski, G. Evaluation of the correlation between IL-1β, IL-8, IFN-γ cytokine concentration in cervico-vaginal fluid and the risk of preterm delivery. *Ginekol. Pol.* **2015**, *86*, 821–826. [CrossRef]
14. Kucukgul, S.; Ozkan, Z.S.; Yavuzkir, S.; Ilhan, N. Investigation of the maternal and cord plasma levels of IL-1 beta, TNF-alpha and VEGF in early membrane rupture. *Matern. Fetal Neonatal Med.* **2016**, *29*, 2157–2160. [CrossRef]
15. Vadillo-Ortega, F.; Estrada-Gutierrez, G. Role of matrix metalloproteinases in preterm labour. *BJOG An Int. J. Obstet. Gynaecol.* **2005**, *112* (Suppl. 1), 19–22. [CrossRef] [PubMed]
16. Campbell, S. Universal cervical-length screening and vaginal progesterone prevents early preterm births, reduces neonatal morbidity and is cost saving: Doing nothing is no longer an option. *Ultrasound Obstet. Gynecol.* **2011**, *38*, 1–9. [CrossRef] [PubMed]
17. Kagan, K.O.; To, M.; Tsoi, E.; Nicolaides, K.H. Preterm birth: The value of sonographic measurement of cervical length. *BJOG* **2006**, *113* (Suppl. 3), 52–56. [CrossRef] [PubMed]
18. Ophir, J.; Cespedes, I.; Ponnekanti, H.; Yazdi, Y.; Li, X. Elastography: A quantitative method for imaging the elasticity of biological tissues. *Ultrason. Imaging* **1991**, *13*, 111–134. [CrossRef] [PubMed]
19. Forroro, L.; Selvatat, J.P.; Bonard, J.M.; Bacsa, R.; Thomson, N.H.; Garaj, S.; Thien-Nga, L.; Gaal, R.; Kulik, A.; Ruzicka, B.; et al. Electronic and Mechanical Properties of Carbon Nanotubes. Available online: https://link.springer.com/content/pdf/10.1007/0-306-47098-5_22.pdf (accessed on 1 January 2002).
20. Albayrak, E.; Dogru, H.Y.; Ozmen, Z.; Altunkas, A.; Kalayci, T.O.; Inci, M.F.; Server, S.; Sonmezgoz, F.; Aktas, F.; Demir, O. Is evaluation of placenta with real-time sonoelastography during the second trimester of pregnancy an effective method for the assessment of spontaneous preterm birth risk? *Clin. Imaging* **2016**, *40*, 926–930. [CrossRef]
21. Agrez, M.; Gu, X.; Giles, W. Matrix metalloproteinase 9 activity in urine of patients at risk for premature delivery. *Am. J. Obstet. Gynecol.* **1999**, *181*, 387–388. [CrossRef]
22. Balbin, M.; Fueyo, A.; Knauper, V.; Pendás, A.M.; López, J.M.; Jiménez, M.G.; Murphy, G.; López-Otín, C. Collagenase 2 (MMP-8) expression in murine tissue-remodeling processes. Analysis of its potential role in postpartum involution of the uterus. *J. Biol. Chem.* **1998**, *273*, 23959–23968. [CrossRef]
23. Iams, J.D. Prediction and early detection of preterm labour. *Obstet. Gynecol.* **2003**, *101*, 402–412. [PubMed]
24. Mercer, B.M. Preterm premature rupture of the membranes. *Obstet. Gynecol.* **2003**, *101*, 178–193. [PubMed]
25. Nien, J.K.; Yoon, B.H.; Espinoza, J.; Kusanovic, J.P.; Erez, O.; Soto, E.; Richani, K.; Gomez, R.; Hassan, S.; Mazor, M.; et al. A rapid MMP-8 bedside test for the detection of intra-amniotic inflammation identifies patients at risk for imminent preterm delivery. *Am. J. Obstet. Gynecol.* **2006**, *195*, 1025–1030. [CrossRef]
26. Cooper, L.G.; Leland, N.L.; Alexander, G. Effect of maternal age on birth outcomes among young adolescents. *Soc. Biol.* **1995**, *42*, 22–35. [CrossRef]
27. Reichman, N.E.; Pagnini, D.L. Maternal age and birth outcomes: Data from New Jersey. *Fam. Plann. Perspect.* **1997**, *29*, 268–272, 295. [CrossRef] [PubMed]
28. Astolfi, P.; De Pasquale, A.; Zonta, L. Late childbearing and its impact on adverse pregnancy outcome: Stillbirth, preterm delivery and low birth weight. *Rev. Epidemiol. Sante Publique* **2005**, *53*, 97–105. [CrossRef]
29. Berghella, V.; Palacio, M.; Ness, A.; Alfirevic, Z.; Nicolaides, K.H.; Saccone, G. Cervical length screening for prevention of preterm birth in singleton pregnancy with threatened preterm labor: Systematic review and meta-analysis of randomized controlled trials using individual patient-level data. *Ultrasound Obstet. Gynecol.* **2017**, *49*, 322–329. [CrossRef]
30. Ville, Y.; Rozenberg, P. Predictors of preterm birth. *Best Pract. Res. Clin. Obstet. Gynaecol.* **2018**, *52*, 23–32. [CrossRef]
31. Greco, E.; Gupta, R.; Syngelaki, A.; Poon, L.C.; Nicolaides, K.H. First-trimester screening for spontaneous preterm delivery with maternal characteristics and cervical length. *Fetal Diagn. Ther.* **2012**, *31*, 154–161. [CrossRef]
32. Andrade, K.C.; Bortoletto, T.G.; Almeida, C.M.; Daniel, R.A.; Avo, H.; Pacagnella, R.C.; Cecatti, J.G. Reference Ranges for Ultrasonographic Measurements of the Uterine Cervix in Low-Risk Pregnant Women. *Rev. Bras. Ginecol. Obstet.* **2017**, *39*, 443–452. [CrossRef]
33. Sharvit, M.; Weiss, R.; Ganor Paz, Y.; Geffen, K.T.; Miller, N.D.; Biron-Shental, T. Vaginal examination vs. cervical length—Which is superior in predicting preterm birth? *J. Perinat. Med.* **2017**, *45*, 977–983. [CrossRef]
34. Molina, F.S.; Gomez, L.F.; Florido, J.; Padilla, M.C.; Nicolaides, K.H. Quantification of cervical elastography: A reproducibility study. *Ultrasound Obstet. Gynecol.* **2012**, *39*, 685–689. [CrossRef]
35. Mazza, E.; Parra-Saavedra, M.; Bajka, M.; Gratacos, E.; Nicolaides, K.; Deprest, J. In vivo assessment of the biomechanical properties of the uterine cervix in pregnancy. *Prenat. Diagn.* **2014**, *34*, 33–41. [CrossRef] [PubMed]
36. Pedretti, M.K.; Kazemier, B.M.; Dickinson, J.E.; Mol, B.W. Implementing universal cervical length screening in asymptomatic women with singleton pregnancies: Challenges and opportunities. *J. Obstet. Gynaecol.* **2017**, *57*, 221–227. [CrossRef] [PubMed]

37. Thomas, A.; Kummel, S.; Gemeinhardt, O.; Fischer, T. Real-time sonoelastography of the cervix: Tissue elasticity of the normal and abnormal cervix. *Acad. Radiol.* **2007**, *14*, 193–200. [CrossRef] [PubMed]
38. Maurer, M.M.; Badir, S.; Pensalfini, M.; Bajka, M.; Abitabile, P.; Zimmermann, R.; Mazza, E. Challenging the in vivo assessment of biomechanical properties of the uterine cervix: A critical analysis of ultrasound based quasi-static procedures. *J. Biomech.* **2015**, *48*, 1541–1548. [CrossRef]
39. Fruscalzo, A.; Schmitz, R.; Klockenbusch, W.; Steinhard, J. Reliability of cervix elastography in late first and second trimester of pregnancy. *Ultraschall Med.* **2012**, *33*, 1–7. [CrossRef] [PubMed]
40. Fruscalzo, A.; Schmitz, R. Quantitative cervical elastography in pregnancy. *Ultra Obstet. Gynecol.* **2012**, *40*, 612. [CrossRef]
41. Parra-Saavedra, M.; Gomez, L.; Barrero, A.; Parra, G.; Vergara, F.; Navarro, E. Prediction of preterm birth using the cervical consistency index. *Ultra Obstet. Gynecol.* **2011**, *38*, 44–51. [CrossRef] [PubMed]
42. Woźniak, S.; Czuczwar, P.; Szkodziak, P.; Wrona, W.; Paszkowski, T. Elastography for predicting preterm delivery in patients with short cervical length at 18–22 weeks of gestation: A prospective observational study. *Ginekol. Pol.* **2015**, *86*, 442–447. [CrossRef]
43. Świątkowska-Freund, M.; Preis, K. Cervical elastography during pregnancy: Clinical perspectives. *Int. J. Womens Health* **2017**, *9*, 245–254. [CrossRef] [PubMed]
44. Pizzella, S.; El Helou, N.; Chubiz, J.; Wang, L.V.; Tuuli, M.G.; England, S.K.; Stout, M.J. Evolving cervical imaging technologies to predict preterm birth. *Semin. Immunopathol.* **2020**, *42*, 385–396. [CrossRef] [PubMed]
45. Pandey, M.; Awasthi, S. Role of MMP-1, MMP-8 and MMP-9 gene polymorphisms in preterm birth. *J. Genet.* **2020**, *99*, 2. [CrossRef]
46. Lee, S.M.; Park, K.H.; Jung, E.Y.; Cho, S.H.; Ryu, A. Prediction of spontaneous preterm birth in women with cervical insufficiency: Comprehensive analysis of multiple proteins in amniotic fluid. *J. Obstet. Gynaecol. Res.* **2016**, *42*, 776–783. [CrossRef] [PubMed]
47. Park, J.W.; Park, K.H.; Jung, E.Y. Clinical significance of histologic chorioamnionitis with a negative amniotic fluid culture in patients with preterm labor and premature membrane rupture. *PLoS ONE* **2017**, *12*, e0173312. [CrossRef]
48. Yoo, H.N.; Park, K.H.; Jung, E.Y.; Kim, Y.M.; Kook, S.Y.; Jeon, S.J. Non-invasive prediction of preterm birth in women with cervical insufficiency or an asymptomatic short cervix (≤25 mm) by measurement of biomarkers in the cervicovaginal fluid. *PLoS ONE* **2017**, *12*, e0180878. Available online: http://journals.plos.org/plosone/article?id=10.1371/journal.pone.0180878 (accessed on 10 July 2017).
49. Becher, N.; Hein, M.; Danielsen, C.C.; Uldbjerg, N. Matrix metalloproteinases in the cervical mucus plug in relation to gestational age, plug compartment, and preterm labor. *Reprod. Biol. Endocrinol.* **2010**, *8*, 113. [CrossRef] [PubMed]
50. Rahkonen, L.; Rutanen, E.M.; Nuutila, M.; Sainio, S.; Sorsa, T.; Paavonen, J. Matrix metalloproteinase-8 in cervical fluid in early and mid pregnancy: Relation to spontaneouspreterm delivery. *Prenat. Diagn.* **2010**, *30*, 1079–1085. [CrossRef]
51. Kuć, P.; Lemancewicz, A.; Laudański, P.; Krętowska, M.; Laudański, T. Total matrix metalloproteinase-8 serum levels in patients labouring preterm and patients with threatened preterm delivery. *Folia Histochem. Cytobiol.* **2010**, *48*, 366–370. [CrossRef]
52. Athayde, N.; Romero, R.; Gomez, R.; Maymon, E.; Pacora, P.; Mazor, M.; Yoon, B.H.; Fortunato, S.; Menon, R.; Ghezzi, F.; et al. Matrix metalloproteinaes-9 in preterm and term human parturition. *J. Matern. Fetal Med.* **1999**, *8*, 213–219.
53. Myntti, T.; Rahkonen, L.; Nupponen, I.; Pätäri-Sampo, A.; Tikkanen, M.; Sorsa, T.; Juhila, J.; Andersson, S.; Paavonen, J.; Stefanovic, V. Amniotic Fluid Infection in Preterm Pregnancies with Intact Membranes. *Dis. Markers* **2017**, *2017*, 1–9. [CrossRef] [PubMed]

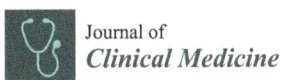

Article

Maternal Systemic Lupus Erythematosus (SLE) High Risk for Preterm Delivery and Not for Long-Term Neurological Morbidity of the Offspring

Dora Davidov [1], Eyal Sheiner [1,*], Tamar Wainstock [2], Shayna Miodownik [1] and Gali Pariente [1]

[1] Soroka University Medical Center, Department of Obstetrics and Gynecology, Ben-Gurion University of the Negev, Beer-Sheva 84101, Israel; davidora88@gmail.com (D.D.); miodowni@post.bgu.ac.il (S.M.); galipa@bgu.ac.il (G.P.)

[2] The Department of Public Health, Faculty of Health Sciences, Ben-Gurion University of the Negev, Beer-Sheva 84101, Israel; wainstoc@post.bgu.ac.il

* Correspondence: sheiner@bgu.ac.il

Abstract: Objective: Pregnancies of women with systemic lupus erythematosus (SLE) are associated with preterm delivery. As preterm delivery is associated with long-term neurological morbidity, we opted to evaluate the long-term neurologic outcomes of offspring born to mothers with SLE regardless of gestational age. Methods: Perinatal outcomes and long-term neurological disease of children of women with and without SLE during pregnancy were evaluated. Children of women with and without SLE were followed until 18 years of age for neurological diseases. Generalized estimating equation (GEE) models were used to assess perinatal outcomes. To compare cumulative neurological morbidity incidence a Kaplan–Meier survival curve was used, and a Cox proportional hazards model was used to control for confounders. Result: A total of 243,682 deliveries were included, of which 100 (0.041%) were of women with SLE. Using a GEE model, maternal SLE was noted as an independent risk factor for preterm delivery. The cumulative incidence of long-term neurological disease was not found to be significantly higher when using the Kaplan Meier survival curves and maternal SLE was not found to be associated with long term neurological disease of the offspring when a Cox model was used. Conclusion: Despite the association of SLE with preterm delivery, no difference in long-term neurological disease was found among children of women with or without SLE.

Keywords: systemic lupus erythematosus; preterm delivery; neurologic morbidity; offspring

1. Introduction

Systemic lupus erythematosus (SLE) is a chronic multisystemic autoimmune inflammatory disease with a wide range of clinical manifestations and it affects many organ systems [1]. While SLE mainly affects young women of childbearing age, the prevalence varies with the sex, age and ethnicity [1–3]. Treatment of SLE focuses on preventing and decreasing the severity and duration of flares, with the use of NSAIDs and antimalarial drugs for mild to moderate SLE and high dose corticosteroids for severe disease [4,5].

Antiphospholipid antibodies (aPL) are the main predictors of pregnancy complications, including miscarriage, fetal death, prematurity and preeclampsia, with lupus anticoagulant (LAC) being strongly associated with miscarriage and late fetal loss [6–8]. Furthermore, infants of mothers with SLE who were exposed to anti-Ro/SSA or anti-La/SSB antibodies during pregnancy have shown an increased risk for neonatal lupus syndrome, with its most serious manifestation being fetal heart block [6,9,10].

Previous studies have examined immediate pregnancy outcomes of women with SLE. Recurrent pregnancy loss, preeclampsia, fetal growth restriction, preterm delivery, cesarean delivery and postpartum infections [9,11,12] are some of the obstetrical complications shown to be correlated with SLE.

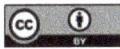

Studies have pointed out an association of long-term neurological diseases in children of mothers with SLE, such as neurodevelopment impairment, learning and speech disorder, attention deficit hyperactivity disorder (ADHD) and autism spectrum disorders [13–15]. However these studies were limited by smaller cohorts.

Several factors have been suggested to affect neurodevelopment impairment among children born to mothers with SLE. This largely involves maternal autoantibodies that cross the placenta during fetal development which may result in learning disorders and dyslexia in offspring [16,17]. Additionally, prematurity was found to be linked to long-term neurological disease, such as cerebral palsy, particularly when chorioamnionitis was involved [18,19].

Due to the link between maternal SLE and preterm delivery, we opted to investigate the association between maternal SLE and unfavorable perinatal outcome, and long term neurological disease of children born to mothers with SLE, regardless of gestational age.

2. Materials and Methods

This was a population-based retrospective cohort study that investigated perinatal results and long-term neurological diseases of children of mothers with and without SLE. The study compared various perinatal outcomes, such as perinatal mortality, caesarean delivery, recurrent pregnancy loss, hypertensive disorders, placental abruption and preterm delivery. A predefined set of ICD-9 codes (Table S1) was used as the basis for assessing the total neurological diseases of children of mothers with SLE up to the age of 18 years. These neurological diseases included psychiatric emotional disorders, movement disorders and total neurologic-related hospitalizations. Follow-up time was determined as time to an event (hospitalization with any neurological diagnosis). If any of the following occurred, follow-up ended: hospitalization resulting in death, first hospitalization with any neurological diagnosis or when the child reached 18 years of age. The study population included all children born to mothers with SLE during the years 1991–2014 at Soroka University Medical Center (SUMC), a tertiary hospital and the only medical center in the Negev, the southern region of the country, which covers 65% of the country's area (about 1.22 million people) [20]. Multifetal pregnancies and cases of congenital anomalies and chromosomal abnormalities were excluded from the study. Cases of perinatal mortality were excluded from the long-term analysis. Pregnancies prior or after the study period (1991–2014) were not included in the study. Hence some of the women in our study were multipara but only part of their pregnancies was included in our study. The institutional review board, in accordance with Helsinki declaration, approved the study (IRB number 0357-19-SOR).

Data were collected from two cross-linked and merged computerized databases, each based on mother and infant ID numbers: the perinatal database of the Obstetrics and Gynecology Department and the pediatric hospitalization database of SUMC (Demog-ICD9). The perinatal database contains maternal demographics, diseases and perinatal results documented immediately after delivery and anonymized before analysis. The pediatric hospitalization database contains demographic data and ICD-9 codes for all medical diagnoses recorded during any hospitalization at SUMC.

Among 100 women with SLE, data regarding disease activity, manifestations, presence of anti-Ro/La antibodies, anti dsDNA antibodies and anti-phospholipid syndrome (APS) antibodies were gathered by examining each women's file. The data were in 70% of the files (i.e., 30 women with SLE did not have information regarding disease activity or lack thereof during pregnancy). Severe SLE during pregnancy was defined as having active SLE during pregnancy (i.e., experiencing any SLE manifestation during pregnancy).

Statistical Analysis

Statistical analysis was executed utilizing SPSS 23rd edition. To compare background characteristics between the two study groups, univariable analysis was performed which included *t*-tests or Mann-Whitney U tests for continuous variables and chi-square tests for categorical variables. Generalized estimating equation (GEE) models were used to compare perinatal outcomes, controlling for confounders and for maternal clusters. To compare the cumulative incidence of neurologic-related hospitalization in offspring of mothers with and without SLE a Kaplan-Meier survival curve was used. Finally, a Cox proportional hazards model was used to control for confounders. A p-value of ≤ 0.05 was considered statistically significant. All analyses were two-sided.

Based on initial analysis, after excluding the offspring who did not meet the inclusion criteria, there were 242,246 offspring born to mothers without SLE, and 96 offspring born to mothers with SLE. The rate of pediatric neurological-associated hospitalizations, based on initial analysis, was 4.2% ($n = 4x$). This sample size has a power of 80% to detect an odds ratio of 5.8% between the study groups.

3. Results

3.1. Maternal Characteristics and Perinatal Outcomes

This study included 243,682 deliveries that met the inclusion criteria, of which 100 were from women with SLE (0.041%). Information regarding disease activity during pregnancy was found in 70 women with SLE, of those, 20 women had flares during pregnancy. Disease activity manifested with arthritis (12 women), nephritis (9 women), dermatitis (8 women) and carditis (1 woman). Some women with flares had more than one clinical manifestation. While anti Ro/La antibodies were present in 3 women with flares during pregnancy, anti dsDNA antibodies were present in 10 women with SLE flares during pregnancy. Two women had prior APS antibodies. No information regarding prior organ damage was found in our population. Demographic and clinical characteristics of women with SLE are presented in Table 1.

Table 1. Demographic and clinical characteristics of mothers with and without SLE.

Characteristic	Mothers with SLE ($n = 100$)	Mothers without SLE ($n = 243,582$)	Odds Ratio (95% Confidence Interval)	p-Value
Maternal age, years (mean $\pm$ SD)	31.44 $\pm$ 4.62	28.16 $\pm$ 5.8	-	0.001
Gravidity (%)				
1	18.0	19.7		
2–4	23.0	47.8	-	0.585
≥ 5	59.0	32.5		
Parity (%)				
1	24.0	23.6		
2–4	65.0	51.1	-	0.003
≥ 5	11.0	25.3		
Recurrent pregnancy loss (%)	23.0	5.0	5.63 (3.53–8.98)	<0.001

Mothers with SLE were older and demonstrated higher rates of recurrent pregnancy loss. Perinatal outcomes of the study population are described in Table 2.

Higher rates of hypertensive disorders (13.0% vs. 5.0%, $p < 0.001$ (caesarean delivery (40.0% vs. 13.5%, $p < 0.001$), preterm delivery (28.0% vs. 6.9%, $p < 0.001$) and perinatal mortality (4.0% vs. 0.5%, $p < 0.001$) were noted among women with SLE compared with women without SLE.

A GEE model that controlled for maternal age and disorders of hypertension demonstrated that maternal SLE was an independent risk factor for preterm delivery (adjusted OR 4.9, 95% CI 3.20–7.80, $p < 0.001$). Using another GEE model controlling for gestational age, the association between maternal SLE and perinatal mortality lost its significance (adjusted OR 2.4, 95% CI 0.78–7.93, $p = 0.123$, Table 3).

Table 2. Perinatal outcomes of women with and without SLE.

Characteristic	Women with SLE (n = 100) (%)	Women without SLE (n = 243,582) (%)	Odds Ratio	95% CI	p-Value
Hypertensive disorders	13.0	5.0	2.8	1.57–5.06	<0.001
Placental abruption	1.0	0.6	1.8	0.25–12.92	0.552
Preterm delivery	28.0	6.9	5.2	3.41–8.18	<0.001
Caesarean delivery	40.0	13.5	4.2	2.85–6.35	<0.001
1-Min Apgar score <7	8.0	5.3	1.5	0.75–3.18	0.258
5-Min Apgar score <7	3.0	2.3	1.3	0.42–4.22	0.496
Small for gestational age (SGA)	7.0	4.6	1.5	0.71–3.34	0.260
Perinatal mortality	4.0	0.5	7.5	2.77–20.57	<0.001

Table 3. GEE models for preterm delivery and perinatal mortality.

	Outcome		Adjusted OR	95% CI	p-Value
Model 1 *	Preterm Delivery	Maternal SLE (vs. no maternal SLE)	4.9	3.20–7.80	<0.001
Model 2 **	Perinatal mortality	Maternal SLE (vs. no maternal SLE)	2.4	0.78–7.39	0.123

* Model 1 controls for maternal age and hypertensive disorders. ** Model 2 controls for gestational age at birth.

3.2. Long Term Neurological Morbidity of Offspring to Mothers with SLE

After eliminating all cases of antepartum, intrapartum, and postpartum mortality, the population of the study included 242,342 children, among them 96 children of mothers with SLE. No significant difference was noted in long-term neurological disease between children to mothers with SLE and without SLE (4.2% vs. 3.1%, p = 0.552, Table 4).

Table 4. Selected long-term neurological morbidity in offspring of women with and without SLE.

Neurological Morbidity	Maternal SLE (n = 96)	No maternal SLE (n = 242,246)	p-Value
Movement disorder (%)	3.1	1.8	0.351
Psychiatric emotional disorder (%)	1.0	0.5	0.443
Total neurological hospitalizations (%)	4.2	3.1	0.552

Severe SLE during pregnancy was defined as having flares of SLE manifestations during pregnancy. No significant difference was noted in long-term neurological disease between children to mothers with severe SLE during pregnancy compared with children to mothers with SLE with no manifestation of severity during pregnancy (p = 0.79)

Similarly, no significantly higher cumulative incidence rate of long-term neurological morbidity in offspring of women with SLE was demonstrated by the Kaplan Meier survival curve (log-rank test p = 0.429, Figure 1).

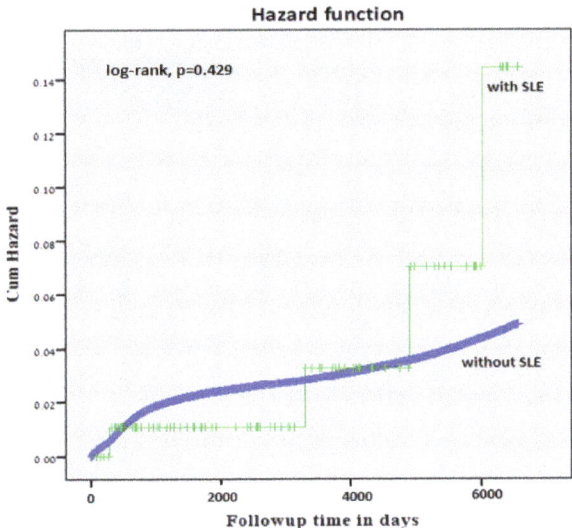

Figure 1. Kaplan-Meier survival curve demonstrating the cumulative incidence of neurologic-related hospitalizations in offspring of mothers with and without SLE (log-rank test, $p = 0.429$).

A Cox proportional hazards model, controlling for gestational age and maternal age, demonstrated that being born to a mother with SLE was not found to be independently associated with long-term neurological disease of the offspring (adjusted HR 1.3, 95% CI 0.51–3.62, $p = 0.539$, Table 5).

Table 5. Long-term neurological morbidity of children to women with SLE assessed by Cox proportional hazards model.

	Adjusted HR	95% CI	p Value
Maternal SLE (vs. no maternal SLE)	1.3	0.51–3.62	0.539
Preterm delivery (<37 weeks)	1.5	1.41–1.65	<0.001
Mother Age at Birth	0.9	0.99–1.00	0.268

4. Discussion

The major finding of our study is that while maternal SLE was associated with a significantly higher risk for adverse perinatal outcomes such as preterm delivery, no significant difference in long-term neurological morbidity was found between offspring born to mothers with or without SLE.

4.1. Perinatal Outcomes of Mothers with SLE

The association between maternal SLE and adverse perinatal outcomes is well established. Studies of perinatal outcomes in women with SLE showed higher rates of recurrent pregnancy loss, preeclampsia, fetal growth restriction, cesarean delivery, postpartum infections and preterm delivery [12,21].

Our study supports these findings, as hypertensive disorders, cesarean delivery rates, and recurrent pregnancy loss were higher among mothers with SLE compered with mothers without SLE. Preterm delivery rates were also higher among mothers with SLE. As preterm delivery has been demonstrated to be associated with maternal age [22], and hypertensive disorders [23,24], after using a GEE model controlling for maternal age and hypertensive disorders, maternal SLE was independently associated with preterm delivery.

4.2. Long Term Neurological Morbidity in Offspring Born to Mothers with SLE

Contrary to our study, previous studies found an increased risk for long-term neurological morbidity in offspring of mothers with SLE, including learning disorders, ADHD and autism spectrum disorders [14,16,25,26]. Nalli, et al. [26] reported an increased risk of learning disorders in offspring to mothers positive for aPL antibodies. Nevertheless, a restricted sample size of only 10 children born to mothers with SLE, lack of a control group such as children born to mothers with systemic autoimmune diseases yet negative for aPL and self reported evaluations made it hard to interpret the study results. In their case-control study, Ross, et al. [16] studied 58 children born to mothers with SLE and 58 children born to healthy mothers. The authors demonstrated that sons of women with SLE, rather than daughters, were significantly more likely to have learning disabilities, and that the presence of anti-Ro and anti-La antibodies and disease activity were significantly related to a higher prevalence of learning disabilities in the offspring. As our study focused on neurological morbidity that is related to the health of the offspring, learning disabilities were not addressed in our study.

Prior studies have demonstrated the influence of maternal autoantibodies on several aspects of fetal development during pregnancy, such as the presence of anti-Ro/anti-La antibodies and the increased risk of neonatal lupus and congenital heart block [13,17,27]. Other studies indicated that anti-La antibodies were associated with developmental delays in offspring [26,28].

Animal studies demonstrated that anti-dsDNA antibodies and anti-NMDR antibodies, which are both present in SLE patients, cross the placenta and influence fetal neurological development [29]. Surprisingly, our study did not demonstrate a significant association between maternal SLE and long-term neurological morbidity. Lack of association might be due to the fact that some neurological-related morbidities only manifest at ages older than 18 years. Another explanation may be related to the fact that most women with SLE in our population did not manifest symptoms of severe disease during pregnancy and only a minority had positive autoantibodies such as anti-Ro/La of dsDNA autoantibodies. To understand the association between maternal SLE and its long-term neurological effects on offspring, further studies should be done to assess the neurodevelopment spectrum of offspring from childhood to adolescence and differences in offspring outcome between women with and without severe SLE during pregnancy.

4.3. Strengths and Limitations of the Study

Our study worked with a large population and with a long follow-up period, in an effort to evaluate the risk of neurologic-related hospitalizations in children born to mothers with SLE, thereby decreasing the chances of incorrect exposure and outcome data. By combining maternal, neonatal, and long-term childhood data, we were able to demonstrate the long-term outcomes of children, while controlling for several parameters during pregnancy and delivery. Healthcare in the country is universal, with all citizens provided equal and free medical care irrespective of their socio-economic standing. Inequity in medical access being reduced in such circumstances, it is unlikely that differences between social classes would be encountered. Nevertheless, our study has several limitations. First, our study lacked some clinical data regarding the severity of the disease, presence of specific antibodies and the treatment that was provided to mothers with SLE. However, as the two most common medications for treatment of SLE include antimalarial agents and corticosteroids, which have not been shown to effect long-term neurological development of the offspring, we would assume that the treatment provided to the mother would not influence the study's results [30–34]. In addition to this no data regarding the reasons for the preterm deliveries or the reasons for the perinatal mortality cases were known to us, Secondly, because our study was based on hospitalizations alone, our data include only severe neurological morbidities and exclude minor morbidities that are mainly treated in regional clinics. Another limitation of our study is the rareness of both the exposure (maternal SLE) and outcome (long- term neurological morbidity of the offspring) in our population, which may result in lack of power to demonstrate a positive correlation between the two. Finally, since patients can choose other places of health care, patients may have chosen to be treated in health centers other than SUMC

5. Conclusions

In conclusion, in our study population, maternal SLE does not appear to increase the risk for long-term neurologic hospitalizations in offspring. As most women with SLE during pregnancy in our population did not have severe disease during pregnancy and as the activity of the disease may influence the association between maternal SLE and long-term morbidity of the offspring, additional studies should investigate differences between mild to severe maternal SLE and their association with long- term neurological morbidity of the offspring. Further studies should also investigate the association between maternal SLE and other related neurodevelopmental concerns, in order to identify populations at need for long-term surveillance.

Supplementary Materials: The following are available online at https://www.mdpi.com/article/10.3390/jcm10132952/s1, Table S1: neurological morbidities ICD-9 codes.

Author Contributions: Conceptualization, D.D. and G.P.; methodology, T.W.; software, T.W.; validation, T.W.; formal analysis, T.W.; investigation, D.D. and G.P.; resources, G.P.; data curation, T.W.; writing—original draft preparation, D.D.; writing—review and editing, G.P., E.S., and S.M.; visualization, D.D.; supervision, G.P. and E.S.; project administration, G.P. All authors have read and agreed to the published version of the manuscript.

Funding: This research received no external funding.

Conflicts of Interest: The authors declare no conflict of interest.

References

1. Rahman, A.; Isenberg, D. Systemic Lupus Erythematosus. *N. Engl. J. Med.* **2008**, *358*, 929–939. [CrossRef]
2. Dörner, T.; Furie, R. Novel paradigms in systemic lupus erythematosus. *Lancet* **2019**, *393*, 2344–2358. [CrossRef]
3. Rees, F.; Doherty, M.; Grainge, M.; Lanyon, P.; Zhang, W. The worldwide incidence and prevalence of systemic lupus erythematosus: A systematic review of epidemiological studies. *Rheumatology* **2017**, *56*, 1945–1961. [CrossRef] [PubMed]
4. Wallace, D.J.; Gudsoorkar, V.S.; Weisman, M.H.; Venuturupalli, S.R. New insights into mechanisms of therapeutic effects of antimalarial agents in SLE. *Nat. Rev. Rheumatol.* **2012**, *8*, 522–533. [CrossRef]
5. Mohamed, A.; Chen, Y.; Wu, H.; Liao, J.; Cheng, B.; Lu, Q. Therapeutic advances in the treatment of SLE. *Int. Immunopharmacol.* **2019**, *72*, 218–223. [CrossRef]
6. Ruiz-Irastorza, G.; Khamashta, M. Lupus and pregnancy: Ten questions and some answers. *Lupus* **2008**, *17*, 416–420. [CrossRef] [PubMed]
7. Xu, J.; Chen, D.; Duan, X.; Li, L.; Tang, Y.; Peng, B. The association between antiphospholipid antibodies and late fetal loss: A systematic review and meta-analysis. *Acta Obstet. Gynecol. Scand.* **2019**, *98*, 1523–1533. [CrossRef]
8. Lockshin, M.D.; Kim, M.; Laskin, C.A.; Guerra, M.M.; Branch, D.W.; Merrill, J.T.; Petri, M.; Porter, T.F.; Sammaritano, L.R.; Stephenson, M.D.; et al. Prediction of adverse pregnancy outcome by the presence of lupus anticoagulant, but not anticardiolipin antibody, in patients with antiphospholipid antibodies. *Arthritis Rheum.* **2012**, *64*, 2311–2318. [CrossRef]
9. Singh, A.G.; Chowdhary, V.R. Pregnancy-related issues in women with systemic lupus erythematosus. *Int. J. Rheum. Dis.* **2014**, *18*, 172–181. [CrossRef] [PubMed]
10. Lateef, A.; Petri, M. Management of pregnancy in systemic lupus erythematosus. *Nat. Rev. Rheumatol.* **2012**, *8*, 710–718. [CrossRef]
11. Sammaritano, L.R. Management of Systemic Lupus Erythematosus during Pregnancy. *Annu. Rev. Med.* **2017**, *68*, 271–285. [CrossRef]
12. Bundhun, P.K.; Soogund, M.Z.S.; Huang, F. Impact of systemic lupus erythematosus on maternal and fetal outcomes following pregnancy: A meta-analysis of studies published between years 2001–2016. *J. Autoimmun.* **2017**, *79*, 17–27. [CrossRef] [PubMed]
13. Skog, A.; Tingström, J.; Salomonsson, S.; Sonesson, S.-E.; Wahren-Herlenius, M. Neurodevelopment in children with and without congenital heart block born to anti-Ro/SSA-positive mothers. *Acta Paediatr.* **2012**, *102*, 40–46. [CrossRef]
14. Vinet, É.; Pineau, C.A.; Clarke, A.E.; Scott, S.; Fombonne, E.; Joseph, L.; Platt, R.W.; Bernatsky, S. Increased Risk of Autism Spectrum Disorders in Children Born to Women with Systemic Lupus Erythematosus: Results from a Large Population-Based Cohort. *Arthritis Rheumatol.* **2015**, *67*, 3201–3208. [CrossRef]
15. Neri, F.; Chimini, L.; Bonomi, F.; Filippini, E.; Motta, M.; Faden, D.; Lojacono, A.; Rebaioli, C.B.; Frassi, M.; Danieli, E.; et al. Neuropsychological development of children born to patients with systemic lupus erythematosus. *Lupus* **2004**, *13*, 805–811. [CrossRef] [PubMed]

16. Ross, G.; Sammaritano, L.; Nass, R.; Lockshin, M. Effects of Mothers' Autoimmune Disease during Pregnancy on Learning Disabilities and Hand Preference in Their Children. *Arch. Pediatr. Adolesc. Med.* **2003**, *157*, 397–402. [CrossRef] [PubMed]
17. Behan, W.M.H.; Behan, P.O.; Geschwind, N. Anti-Ro Antibody in Mothers of Dyslexic Children. *Dev. Med. Child Neurol.* **2008**, *27*, 538–540. [CrossRef]
18. Hirvonen, M.; Ojala, R.; Korhonen, P.; Haataja, P.; Eriksson, K.; Gissler, M.; Luukkaala, T.; Tammela, O. Cerebral Palsy Among Children Born Moderately and Late Preterm. *Pediatrics* **2014**, *134*, e1584–e1593. [CrossRef]
19. Freud, A.; Wainstock, T.; Sheiner, E.; Beloosesky, R.; Fischer, L.; Landau, D.; Walfisch, A. Maternal chorioamnionitis & long term neurological morbidity in the offspring. *Eur. J. Paediatr. Neurol.* **2019**, *23*, 484–490. [CrossRef]
20. Central Bureau of Statistics. Israel in Figures, 2008–2017. [Updated 6 February 2019]. Available online: https://www.cbs.gov.il/he/mediarelease/DocLib/2019/042/01_19_042b.pdf (accessed on 30 June 2021).
21. Pastore, D.E.A.; Costa, M.L.; Surita, F.G. Systemic lupus erythematosus and pregnancy: The challenge of improving antenatal care and outcomes. *Lupus* **2019**, *28*, 1417–1426. [CrossRef]
22. Fuchs, F.; Monet, B.; Ducruet, T.; Chaillet, N.; Audibert, F. Effect of maternal age on the risk of preterm birth: A large cohort study. *PLoS ONE* **2018**, *13*, e0191002. [CrossRef] [PubMed]
23. Heard, A.R.; Dekker, G.A.; Chan, A.; Jacobs, D.J.; Vreeburg, S.A.; Priest, K.R. Hypertension during pregnancy in South Australia, Part 1: Pregnancy outcomes. *Aust. N. Z. J. Obstet. Gynaecol.* **2004**, *44*, 404–409. [CrossRef]
24. Maducolil, M.K.; Al-Obaidly, S.; Olukade, T.; Salama, H.; AlQubaisi, M.; Al Rifai, H. Maternal characteristics and pregnancy outcomes of women with chronic hypertension: A population-based study. *J. Périnat. Med.* **2020**, *48*, 139–143. [CrossRef] [PubMed]
25. Urowitz, M.B.; Gladman, D.D.; MacKinnon, A.; Ibañez, D.; Bruto, V.; Rovet, J.; Silverman, E. Neurocognitive abnormalities in offspring of mothers with systemic lupus erythematosus. *Lupus* **2008**, *17*, 555–560. [CrossRef]
26. Nalli, C.; Iodice, A.; Andreoli, L.; Galli, J.; Lojacono, A.; Motta, M.; Fazzi, E.; Tincani, A. Long-term neurodevelopmental outcome of children born to prospectively followed pregnancies of women with systemic lupus erythematosus and/or antiphospholipid syndrome. *Lupus* **2017**, *26*, 552–558. [CrossRef] [PubMed]
27. Wahren-Herlenius, M.; Sonesson, S.-E. Specificity and effector mechanisms of autoantibodies in congenital heart block. *Curr. Opin. Immunol.* **2006**, *18*, 690–696. [CrossRef] [PubMed]
28. Marder, W.; Romero, V.C.; Ganser, M.A.; Hyzy, M.A.; Gordon, C.; McCune, W.J.; Somers, E.C. Increased usage of special educational services by children born to mothers with systemic lupus erythematosus and antiphospholipid antibodies. *Lupus Sci. Med.* **2014**, *1*, e000034. [CrossRef]
29. Wang, L.; Zhou, D.; Lee, J.; Niu, H.; Faust, T.W.; Frattini, S.; Kowal, C.; Huerta, P.; Volpe, B.T.; Diamond, B. Female mouse fetal loss mediated by maternal autoantibody. *J. Exp. Med.* **2012**, *209*, 1083–1089. [CrossRef] [PubMed]
30. Skuladottir, H.; Wilcox, A.; Ma, C.; Lammer, E.J.; Rasmussen, S.A.; Werler, M.M.; Shaw, G.M.; Carmichael, S.L. Corticosteroid use and risk of orofacial clefts. *Birth Defects Res. Part A Clin. Mol. Teratol.* **2014**, *100*, 499–506. [CrossRef] [PubMed]
31. Van Zutphen, A.R.; Bell, E.M.; Browne, M.L.; Lin, S.; Lin, A.E.; Druschel, C.M.; The National Birth Defects Prevention Study. Maternal asthma medication use during pregnancy and risk of congenital heart defects. *Birth Defects Res. Part A Clin. Mol. Teratol.* **2015**, *103*, 951–961. [CrossRef]
32. Clowse, M.E.B.; Magder, L.; Witter, F.; Petri, M. Hydroxychloroquine in lupus pregnancy. *Arthritis Rheum.* **2006**, *54*, 3640–3647. [CrossRef] [PubMed]
33. Cooper, W.O.; Cheetham, T.C.; Li, D.-K.; Stein, C.M.; Callahan, S.T.; Morgan, T.M.; Shintani, A.K.; Chen, N.; Griffin, M.R.; Ray, W.A. Brief report: Risk of adverse fetal outcomes associated with immunosuppressive medications for chronic immune-mediated diseases in pregnancy. *Arthritis Rheumatol.* **2013**, *66*, 444–450. [CrossRef] [PubMed]
34. Abarientos, C.; Sperber, K.; Shapiro, D.L.; Aronow, W.S.; Chao, C.P.; Ash, J.Y. Hydroxychloroquine in systemic lupus erythematosus and rheumatoid arthritis and its safety in pregnancy. *Expert Opin. Drug Saf.* **2011**, *10*, 705–714. [CrossRef] [PubMed]

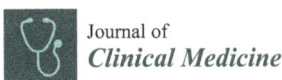

Article

Identifying the Critical Threshold for Long-Term Pediatric Neurological Hospitalizations of the Offspring in Preterm Delivery

Shiran Zer [1], Tamar Wainstock [2], Eyal Sheiner [1,*], Shayna Miodownik [1] and Gali Pariente [1]

1. Department of Obstetrics and Gynecology, Soroka University Medical Center, Ben-Gurion University of the Negev, Beer-Sheva 84101, Israel; prosz1@walla.com (S.Z.); miodowni@post.bgu.ac.il (S.M.); galipa@bgu.ac.il (G.P.)
2. The Department of Public Health, Faculty of Health Sciences, Ben-Gurion University of the Negev, Beer-Sheva 84101, Israel; wainstoc@post.bgu.ac.il
* Correspondence: sheiner@bgu.ac.il; Tel.: +972-5048045074

Abstract: We opted to investigate whether a critical threshold exists for long-term pediatric neurological morbidity, and cerebral palsy (CP), in preterm delivery, via a population-based cohort analysis. Four study groups were classified according to their gestational age at birth: 24–27.6, 28–31.6, 32–36.6 weeks and term deliveries, evaluating the incidence of long-term hospitalizations of the offspring due to neurological morbidity. Cox proportional hazard models were performed to control for confounders. A Kaplan–Meier survival curve was used to compare the cumulative neurological morbidity incidence for each group. A total of 220,563 deliveries were included: 0.1% (118) occurred at 24–27.6 weeks of gestation, 0.4% (776) occurred at 28–31.6 weeks of gestation, 6% (13,308) occurred at 32–36.6 weeks of gestation and 93% (206,361) at term. In a Cox model, while adjusting for confounders, delivery before 25 weeks had a 3.9-fold risk for long-term neurological morbidity (adjusted HR (hazard ratio) = 3.9, 95% CI (confidence interval) 2.3–6.6; $p < 0.001$). The Kaplan–Meier survival curve demonstrated a linear association between long-term neurological morbidity and decreasing gestational age. In a second Cox model, adjusted for confounders, infants born before 25 weeks of gestation had increased rates of CP (adjusted HR = 62.495% CI 25.6–152.4; $p < 0.001$). In our population, the critical cut-off for long-term neurological complications is delivery before 25 weeks gestation.

Keywords: preterm birth; neurological; pediatric

Citation: Zer, S.; Wainstock, T.; Sheiner, E.; Miodownik, S.; Pariente, G. Identifying the Critical Threshold for Long-Term Pediatric Neurological Hospitalizations of the Offspring in Preterm Delivery. *J. Clin. Med.* **2021**, *10*, 2919. https://doi.org/10.3390/jcm10132919

Academic Editors: Michael G. Ross and Emmanuel Andrès

Received: 23 May 2021
Accepted: 28 June 2021
Published: 29 June 2021

Publisher's Note: MDPI stays neutral with regard to jurisdictional claims in published maps and institutional affiliations.

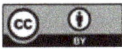

Copyright: © 2021 by the authors. Licensee MDPI, Basel, Switzerland. This article is an open access article distributed under the terms and conditions of the Creative Commons Attribution (CC BY) license (https://creativecommons.org/licenses/by/4.0/).

1. Introduction

Globally, an estimated 15 million infants are born preterm annually [1], and preterm birth (PTB) remains the leading cause of death under the age of 5 years [2]. The World Health Organization (WHO) defines PTB as all births before 37 completed weeks of gestation, with a further sub-division based on gestational age; extremely PTB (delivery at less than 28.0 weeks of gestation), very PTB (delivery between 28.0 and 31.6 weeks of gestation) and moderate to late PTB (delivery between 32.0 and 36.6 weeks of gestation) [1].

Over the past few decades, improvements in modern obstetrics, perinatology, and neonatal care have resulted in an improved survival of the premature infant [3–6]. Among the improvements is included the widespread application of antenatal glucocorticoid therapy, the introduction of synthetic surfactant, and a tendency towards more aggressive feeding strategies [7]. Thus, premature infants are surviving with major and minor neurodevelopmental morbidities, often resulting in lifelong disability [8]. Neurodevelopmental impairments can include, among other morbidities, cerebral palsy (CP), cognitive dysfunction, and sensory impairments [6,9,10].

As the most common cause of severe physical disability in childhood [11,12], CP defines a group of permanent disorders that has occurred in the developing fetal or infant's brain, resulting in severe limitation of activity [12–15]. In CP, motor impairment is often accompanied by disturbances of sensation, perception, cognition, communication and behavior [15]. The overall prevalence of CP is estimated to be 2 per 1000 live births [6,11,16] and its risk is inversely proportional to gestational weight and age at birth, but not necessarily increasing severity [6]. The prevalence of CP expressed by gestational age is reported to be 14.6% in extremely preterm children, 6.2% in very preterm children, and 0.7% in moderate to late preterm compared with 0.11% in term-born children [16,17].

The pathophysiologic mechanisms accounting for the neurodevelopmental disorders in preterm survivors are poorly understood. Perinatal systemic inflammation may sensitize the developing brain to secondary insults and contribute to sustained central nervous system inflammation [18]. Inflammation and related cytokines that can lead to preterm birth may be combined with genetic and epigenetic factors, altering the preterm infant's brain, making it vulnerable to injury [19–22].

As neurologic morbidity is one of the devastating outcomes of prematurity, we elected to investigate the association between the grade of prematurity and long-term neurological morbidity of the offspring, in order to set up a critical cut-off at which the long-term neurological morbidity of the offspring would be higher.

2. Materials and Methods

We conducted a retrospective population-based cohort study, which included all singleton pregnancies in women who delivered between the years 1991 and 2014. The study was conducted at the Soroka University Medical Center (SUMC). The hospital assists the local population by providing obstetrical and pediatric care being the only tertiary medical center in the Negev district. The Negev occupies 60% of the land of Israel, and SUMC serves the entire population of the region (14% of Israel's population, approximately 1,190,000) with a birth rate in the southern region showing a positive trend and continues to grow each year [23].

Thus, this study is based on nonselective population data. The Institutional Review Board (in accordance with the Helsinki declaration) approved the study (IRB #0357-19-SOR).

Four groups were evaluated during the study period, based on gestational age, as followed by the WHO (1); extreme PTB: $24 + 0 - 27 + 6$, very PTB: $28 + 0 - 31 + 6$, moderate to late PTB: $32 + 0 - 36 + 6$ weeks of gestation and term deliveries. Neurological morbidity included hospitalizations up to 18 years of age involving a predefined set of ICD-9 (International Classification of Diseases) codes, as recorded in hospital records. Neurological morbidity encompasses movement disorders, developmental disorders, degenerative disorders, psychiatric disorders, and CP (Table S1). Multiple pregnancy, women with lack of prenatal care, women with chromosomal abnormalities or congenital anomalies, and perinatal mortality cases (intrauterine fetal death, intrapartum death, postpartum death) were excluded from the study. All other deliveries were included in the study.

Follow up was terminated if any of the following occurred: the first hospitalization at SUMC for neurological morbidity, any hospitalization which resulted in death, the child reached 18 years of age, or at the end of the study period.

Data were collected from two computerized clinical data sets: the first, perinatal data from the obstetric and gynecologic department at SUMC, including information that was documented by obstetricians directly following delivery. Subsequently, medical secretaries regularly examine the data before it is entered into the database. After evaluating and crossing the hospital documents with prenatal care records, coding is performed. Maximal completeness and accuracy of the databases is fulfilled with these unique measures. The second is a computerized pediatric hospitalization at SUMC (Demog-ICD-9), which includes both demographic data and medical diagnosis during hospitalization. The two databases were cross-linked and merged based on the patients' ID (mother and child). All diagnoses were classified by the international classification of disease (ICD-9).

Neurological outcomes assessed included hospitalization of the offspring up to 18 years of age due to primary or secondary neurological morbidity, with secondary neurological morbidity defined as hospitalization with neurological morbidity not being the primary diagnosis. These outcomes included at least one diagnosis of the following: movement disorder (including seizures disorders), cerebral palsy (including infantile cerebral palsy unspecified, paraplegia, diplegia of upper limbs, and paralysis unspecified), autism spectrum disorders, eating disorders, psychiatric disease, attention deficit hyperactivity disorder, and developmental disorders. The predefined ICD-9 codes of all diagnoses are detailed in the Supplemental Table (Table S1). In our setting, screening for neurological morbidity is performed at The Institute for Child Development, which provides diagnostic services, treatment, and monitoring for children with developmental disorders from birth to 6 years old. Beyond this age, children diagnosed with developmental disorders are referred to at developmental and neurological clinics at SUMC or in the community. Additionally, the Institute for Child Development has close ties with, and oversees, other ambulatory services. Although diagnoses made at the Institute for Child Development diagnoses are not part of the SUMC hospitalization database, these diagnoses are often recorded as background diagnoses in the database when a child is hospitalized. In Israel, early assessment of developmental disorders routinely takes place at community "Well Baby" centers. If an additional evaluation is required, the children and their families are referred to Child and Family Developmental Centers, where the child is evaluated by a multi-disciplinary care team to ascertain eligibility for service provision. Thus, neurological diagnosis may be captured in the SUMC database when a child is referred for hospitalization by the community clinic. Additionally, the community clinic and SUMC share an online interface, which assists in capturing all diagnoses upon admission.

Statistical Analysis

Univariable analysis was performed to compare background characteristics between the 4 study groups. The univariable analysis included Chi-square tests for categorical variables and ANOVA tests for continuous variables according to their distribution. The incidence of long-term (up to the age of 18 years) hospitalizations of the offspring due to neurological morbidity was evaluated in the four gestational week age groups. Cumulative incidence morbidity rates were compared using a Kaplan–Meier survival curve, with use of the log-rank test to determine significant differences. Cox proportional hazards models were conducted to compare neurological associated hospitalization risk among offspring born preterm (using dummy variables), divided based on gestational age and term offspring (the reference group), while adjusting for length of follow up. The models adjusted for potential confounders based on the univariable analysis and on the clinical importance of the variables. The cox regression for long-term neurological hospitalizations was adjusted for maternal age, diabetes mellitus, hypertensive disorder, cesarean section and child year birth. The cox regression for cerebral palsy was adjusted for maternal age and child year birth. The mothers in the cohort were entered as clusters to account for dependence between siblings. All analysis was performed using SPSS package 23rd edition (IBM, Armonk, NY, USA) as well as the STATA software 12th edition (StataCorp, College Station, TX, USA).

3. Results

During the study period, 220,563 deliveries met the inclusion criteria. Of those, 0.1% (118) occurred at 24–27.6 gestational weeks, 0.4% (776) occurred at 28–31.6 gestational weeks, 6% (13,308) occurred at 32–36.6 gestational weeks and 93% (206,361) were born at term. We did not find any significant obvious trend over the years of the study for distributions of preterm birth.

Table 1 presents the demographic maternal characteristics and immediate perinatal outcomes of the study population according to gestational age at birth. There was no difference in maternal age between the groups. Overall parity increased with increasing gestational age. Rates of smokers were highest among women delivering extreme preterm and decreased with increasing gestational age. As gestational age declined, rates of in-vitro fertilization (IVF) pregnancies and low Apgar scores were higher. Diabetes was more prevalent in women delivered preterm, although not in the group of extremely preterm.

Table 1. Maternal characteristics and immediate perinatal outcomes of the study population according to gestational age at birth.

Characteristics	Extreme PTB (n = 118) (%)	Very PTB (n = 776) (%)	Moderate-Late PTB (n = 13,308) (%)	Term Birth (n = 206,361) (%)	p-Value
Maternal Age, years (mean ± SD)	28.47 ± 6.34	28.36 ± 6.37	28.31 ± 6.24	28.24 ± 5.76	0.482
Gravidity					<0.001
1	29.7	24.5	23.3	20.2	
2–4	46.6	44.8	44.5	48.7	
5+	23.7	30.7	32.1	31.2	
Parity					<0.001
1	38.1	31.4	29.0	24.2	
2–4	48.3	47.7	47.7	52.0	
5+	13.6	20.9	23.3	23.8	
Smokers	4.2	1	1.5	1	<0.001
Fertility treatments					<0.001
In vitro fertilization	3.4	2.6	2.3	1.1	
Ovulation induction	1.7	1.8	1.1	0.8	
Hypertensive disorders *	8.5	19.1	12.9	4.7	<0.001
Maternal diabetes **	0.0	6.2	8.1	5.2	<0.001
Induction of labor	14.3	4	27.3	31.8	<0.001
Type of birth					<0.001
Vaginal delivery	48.3	46.5	67.3	83.9	
Assisted vaginal delivery	0	0.6	1.7	3.3	
Cesarean delivery	51.7	52.8	31.0	12.7	
Small for gestational age (SGA)	3.4	1.8	3.6	4.4	<0.001
Apgar score 1 min < 7	49.2	28.1	10.2	4.1	<0.001
Apgar score 5 min < 7	14.4	6.2	2.5	1.4	<0.001

* Hypertensive disorders include chronic hypertension, gestational hypertension preeclampsia and eclampsia. ** Maternal diabetes includes pre-gestational diabetes and gestational diabetes. PTB, preterm birth; SD, standard deviation.

Table 2 reveals the incidence rate of disease-specific neurologic-related hospitalizations of the child in accordance with gestational age at birth. Offspring born prematurely were subjected to significantly more hospitalizations due to movement disorders, cerebral palsy as well as psychiatric disorders compared to term offspring.

Table 2. Incidence rate of disease-specific hospitalizations according to gestational age at birth.

Neurological Morbidity of the Offspring	Extreme PTB (n = 118) (%)	Very PTB (n = 776) (%)	Moderate-Late PTB (n = 13,308) (%)	Term Birth n= (206,361) (%)	p-Value
Movement disorders	4.2	3.5	2.7	1.8	<0.001
Cerebral palsy	4.2	0.9	0.2	0.1	<0.001
Psychiatric disorders	2.5	0.9	0.7	0.5	<0.001
Developmental disorders	0.8	0.3	0.2	0.1	<0.001
Degenerative disorders	0	0.6	0.1	0.1	<0.001

The Kaplan–Meier survival curve demonstrated a linear association between long-term neurological morbidity and decreasing gestational age (Log-Rank test $p < 0.001$, Figure 1).

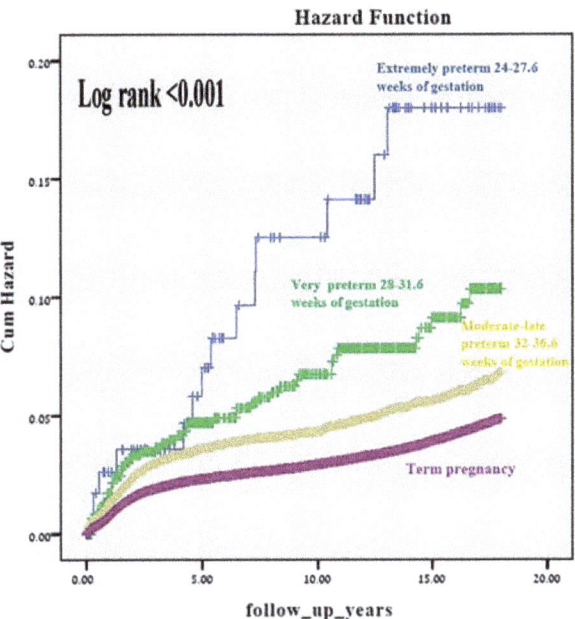

Figure 1. A Kaplan–Meier survival curve exhibiting the cumulative incidence of long-term neurologic-related hospitalizations according to gestational age (Log-Rank test $p < 0.001$).

Figures 2 and 3 represent two Kaplan–Meier curves and each represent the cumulative incidence of long-term neurological hospitalization in two different time periods: 1991–1999 and 2000–2014. No difference in the Log rank test is seen between the two figures.

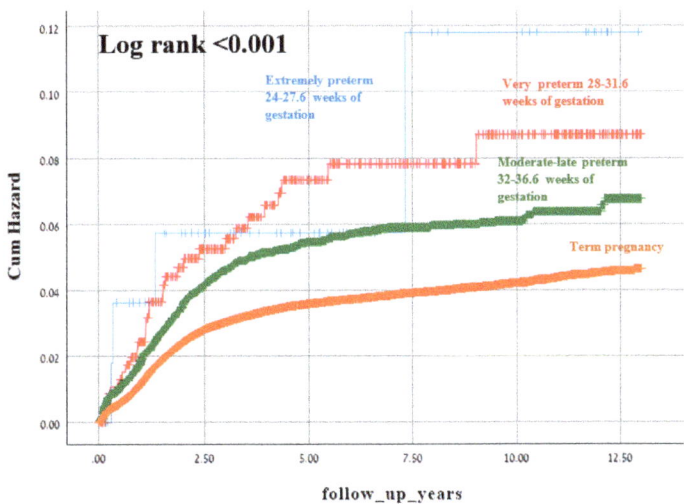

Figure 2. A Kaplan–Meier survival curve demonstrating the cumulative incidence of long-term neurologic-related hospitalizations according to gestational age before year 2000 (Log-Rank test $p < 0.001$).

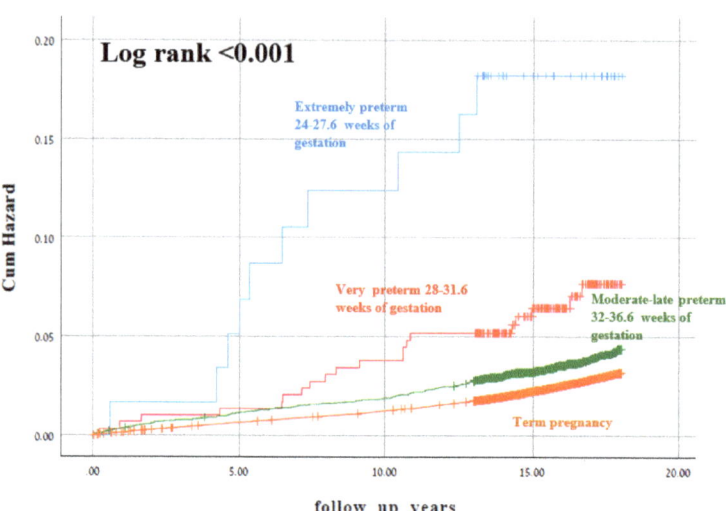

Figure 3. A Kaplan–Meier survival curve demonstrating the cumulative incidence of long-term neurologic-related hospitalizations according to gestational age after year 2000 (Log-Rank test $p < 0.001$).

Figure 4 illustrates univariate analysis of total neurological morbidity according to gestational week at delivery. As seen, the gestational week at birth and neurological morbidity are manifested in an inverse relationship. Searching for a specific threshold, the slope for hospitalization rate attenuated beyond 25 weeks of gestation (Figure 2).

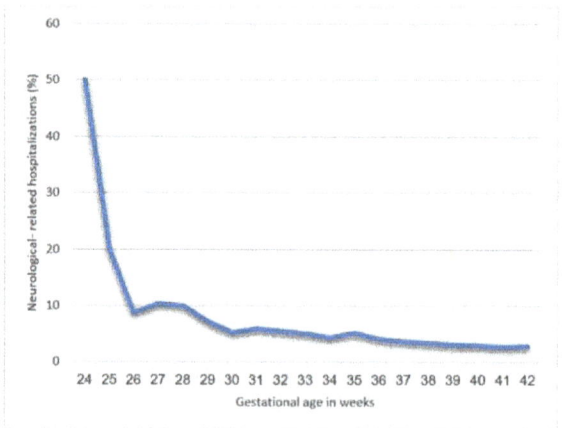

Figure 4. Long-term neurologic-related hospitalizations according to gestational age.

Using a Cox model, adjusting for diabetes, hypertensive disorders and cesarean delivery, delivery before 25 weeks had a 3.9-fold risk for long-term neurological morbidity (adjusted HR = 3.9, 95% CI 2.3–6.6; $p < 0.001$, Table 3). In a second Cox model, which adjusted for maternal age, infants born before 25 weeks of gestation had significantly increased rates of CP (adjusted HR = 62.4, 95% CI 25.6–152.4; $p < 0.001$, Table 3). No differences in the medians of follow-up times were demonstrated between the different gestational ages ($p = 0.179$).

Table 3. Cox multivariable analyses for long-term neurologic-related hospitalizations and for CP according to gestational age.

Gestational Age	Total Neurologic Related Hospitalizations			Cerebral Palsy		
	aHR *	95% CI	p-Value	aHR **	95% CI	p-Value
Term delivery (reference) >37 gestational weeks	1	-	-	1	-	-
Moderate to late preterm	1.3	1.2–1.5	<0.001	2.5	1.6–3.9	<0.001
Very preterm	1.9	1.4–2.5	<0.001	13.4	6.2–28.7	<0.001
Extremely preterm	3.9	2.3–6.6	<0.001	62.4	25.6–152.4	<0.001

* Adjusted for maternal age, diabetes mellitus, hypertensive disorders and cesarean section and childbirth year. ** Adjusted for maternal age and childbirth year. aHR, adjusted hazard ratio, CI, confidence interval.

Table 4 and Figure 5 exhibit Cox proportional hazard models for long-term neurological morbidity according to gestational age. Twenty five weeks is the critical threshold beyond which long-term neurological morbidity decreased. Another reduction of long-term morbidity is seen between 29 and 30 weeks.

Table 4. Cox proportional hazards models for long-term neurological morbidity according to gestational age.

	Gestational Age	Total Neurologic Related Hospitalizations		
		aHR *	95% CI	p-Value
Model 1	PTB 25 gestational week versus other later weeks of PTB	5.9	2.2–15.9	<0.001
Model 2	PTB 26 gestational week versus other later weeks of PTB	2.9	1.4–6.2	<0.004
Model 3	PTB 27 gestational week versus other later weeks of PTB	2.4	1.4–4.2	<0.001
Model 4	PTB 28 gestational week versus other later weeks of PTB	2.3	1.5–3.5	<0.001
Model 5	PTB 29 gestational week versus other later weeks of PTB	2.1	1.4–3.0	<0.001
Model 6	PTB 30 gestational week versus other later weeks of PTB	1.6	1.2–2.2	<0.002
Model 7	PTB 31 gestational week versus other later weeks of PTB	1.5	1.1–1.9	<0.002
Model 8	PTB 32 gestational week versus other later weeks of PTB	1.4	1.1–1.7	<0.003
Model 9	PTB 33 gestational week versus other later weeks of PTB	1.3	1.1–1.6	<0.003
Model 10	PTB 34 gestational week versus other later weeks of PTB	1.2	1.0–1.4	<0.03
Model 11	PTB 35 gestational week versus other later weeks of PTB	1.3	1.1–1.5	<0.001

* Adjusted for maternal age, diabetes mellitus, hypertensive disorders and cesarean section.

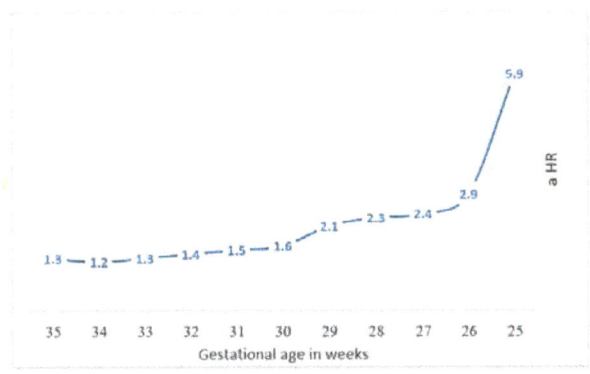

Figure 5. Cox proportional hazard models for long-term neurological morbidity according to gestational age.

4. Discussion

This large retrospective cohort study inspected the long-term incidence of neurologic-related hospitalizations laminated by extremity of prematurity and compared to term offspring. We concluded that decreasing gestational age at birth increased neurological morbidity, as shown in both the Kaplan–Meier survival curve and the Cox regression analysis model. The slope for hospitalization rate according to gestational age attenuated beyond 25 weeks of gestation; therefore, 25 weeks could be determined as the critical threshold below which the risk of neurological morbidity significantly rises, with another threshold effect seen between 29 and 30 weeks, showing a further reduction in long-term neurological morbidity.

These findings are in line with the results of a considerable number of studies in which extremely preterm infants exhibited greater neurodevelopmental impairment than their older gestational age peers [24–26]. Pascal et al., systematic review and meta-analysis demonstrated that overall CP prevalence, along with motor and cognitive delays, were higher in extremely low birthweight infants than in very low birth infants. This variability was only statically significant for CP ($p < 0.001$) and motor delays ($p = 0.012$) [24].

Previous studies from our cohort have investigated the possibility of a critical threshold regarding extremity of prematurity and long-term morbidity of the offspring. A large retrospective population-based study by Davidesko et al. found that children born after 32 weeks gestation were at decreased risk of long-term infectious morbidity [27]. Additionally, Ohana et al. demonstrated a relationship between the degree of prematurity and long-term gastrointestinal morbidity of the offspring, with a critical cut-off at 25 weeks gestation [28].

Studies have indicated that the prevalence of CP among extremely preterm children ranges from 16 to 21% [29]. The EPIPAGE Cohort (étude épidémiologique sur les petits âges gestationnels) study evaluated infants born between 22 and 32 weeks' gestation in nine regions of France in 1997. This study found that at 2 years of age, the prevalence of CP was 20% in those born at 24–26 weeks gestation compared with 4% in those born at 32 weeks [30].

Our study has also demonstrated an independent association between gestational age at birth and the risk for CP. This association may reflect that premature exposure to the extra-uterine environment, including gravity and sensory experiences, can alter musculoskeletal and nervous system development, thereby shifting the trajectory of motor development for otherwise healthy children [26]. Higher rates of CP in the preterm population study groups could be explained by reductions in the rates of post-term births and/or improvements in the accuracy of pregnancy dating over the last decades could have influenced the outcomes of the study.

The human brain develops and matures during the fetal period and is controlled by a set of complex relations among various signaling receptors, genetic/epigenetic factors as well as environmental influences. During the gestational period, several stages of development have been marked: primary neurulation (weeks 3–4), prosencephalic development (months 2–3), neuronal proliferation (months 3–4), neuronal migration (months 3–5), neuronal organization (5 months postnatal period), and myelination. The process of myelination of the human brain spreads from the fetal second trimester and continues postnatally into adulthood, with the quickest growth striking in the immediate neonatal period [31]. The preterm brain is particularly vulnerable because it is exposed to the extra-uterine environment during critical periods of brain development, and is thus at risk of alterations to the "normal" trajectory of brain development [13].

The etiology of neurodevelopmental morbidity, including CP, remains unclear but is thought to be multifactorial. There is increasing evidence that intrauterine or early postnatal inflammation may play a role in the development of CP [32]. Bountiful literature has identified in utero microbial infection and/or inflammation as a strong risk factor for PTB, particularly early spontaneous PTB [33]. The theory is that maternal infection and/or inflammation, occurring during critical periods of fetal development, could alter brain structure and function in a time-sensitive manner, as evidenced by different types of studies. Specifically, in humans, both bacterial and viral infections are associated with abnormal brain structure in affected individuals, while bacterial infections during gestation have been weakly associated with abnormal psychological and cognitive development in their offspring. Data gathered from animal models and retrospective human data and findings advocate potential causative mechanisms for the correlation between injury to the fetal brain and infection; specifically, the inflammatory cascade, caused by infection, is characterized by elevations in various cytokines, such as IL-6, eventually ensuing altered brain structure and function [34].

Amongst the strengths of our study is the population-based nature of its data, and the fact that our hospital serves as only a tertiary medical center of the entire southern region. As a consequence, the majority of the patients are provided with health care services in our facility. The robustness of our conclusions relies on the population-based nature of the cohort, without a selection bias. In our study, vast inclusion criteria and limited exclusion criteria yielded a representative study population. Nevertheless, various limitations in our results should be addressed. The retrospective nature of the data, which are based on a database registry, which has intrinsic limitations related to the type of retrieved information as well as the possibility of misclassification of the outcome (neurological morbidity), provide a major limitation. Most of the neurological conditions evaluated in this study are routinely diagnosed and treated in an ambulatory setting. Thus, our hospital-based database may not reflect the true population morbidity, and some cases will be missed unless the child is hospitalized for any reason. Furthermore, in the case of several of the neurological outcomes, diagnosis is performed via specialized screening. It is therefore possible that there are patients who have the disorder but have not ever been screened. These factors put our study at risk of selection bias. Nevertheless, because some of the conditions included in the study are associated with significant health burdens and comorbidities, sufferers are likely to be hospitalized at one time or another.

Deviation of the results toward the null hypothesis could be caused by this bias. Merely grave neurological morbidities, leading to hospitalizations, were identified, and classified as such. Thus, our conclusions must be restricted to such cases. Even though the southern region is usually influenced by positive immigration, the possibility of immigration of children born outside the hospital coverage zone remains. Another important limitation relates to the study follow-up of the offspring, until the child reaches 18 years old. Various morbidities could arise only at an older age. This deserves to be investigated in future studies. In addition, data regarding interventions to improve perinatal outcomes of preterm infants, including GBS prophylaxis, use of corticosteroids for lung maturation, as well as neuroprotection with magnesium sulfate, were not available for further statistical analysis.

5. Conclusions

In conclusion, very preterm offspring have the highest risk for CP and long-term neurological morbidity. A crucial threshold of 25 weeks gestation was prominent in our study, below which the jeopardy of long-term neurological morbidity of the offspring increased significantly. It is also emphasized that each additional week of gestation further decreased the risk of long-term neurological morbidity, stressing the necessity to consider to properly schedule medically indicated preterm delivery and even early-term delivery in respect of the long-term health of the offspring. Clinical practice should attempt prevention of preterm delivery where possible and attempt to optimize the timing of medically indicted induced delivery as close to full term as medically possible without surpassing an unacceptable increase in the risk to both mother and fetus. Increased surveillance during childhood for signs of neurological impairment could contribute to offspring born prematurely, which is unique for those who born prior to 25 weeks of completed gestation. The mechanisms by which in utero events impact brain injury resulting in subsequent adverse neurodevelopment are extraordinarily complex. Understanding the pathways that lead to observed associations is a challenge that will require immense ongoing scientific rigor.

Supplementary Materials: The following are available online at https://www.mdpi.com/article/10.3390/jcm10132919/s1, Table S1: ICD-9 codes of neurological disorders considered in the study.

Author Contributions: The first two authors equally contributed to the manuscript. Conceptualization, E.S. and G.P.; Formal analysis, T.W.; Methodology, T.W.; Project administration, G.P.; Software, T.W.; Supervision, E.S. and G.P.; Writing—original draft, S.Z.; Writing—review and editing, T.W., E.S. and S.M. All authors have read and agreed to the published version of the manuscript.

Funding: This research received no external funding.

Institutional Review Board Statement: The study was conducted according to the guidelines of the Declaration of Helsinki, and approved by the Institutional Review Board of Soroka university medical center (IRB #0357-19-SOR, approved on 11 December 2019).

Informed Consent Statement: Not applicable.

Data Availability Statement: Due to IRB terms supporting data not provided.

Conflicts of Interest: The authors declare no conflict of interest.

References

1. WHO. Born Too Soon: The Global Action Report on Preterm Birth. Available online: http://www.who.int/pmnch/media/news/2012/preterm_birth_report/en/ (accessed on 23 May 2021).
2. Liu, L.; Oza, S.; Hogan, D.; Perin, J.; Rudan, I.; Lawn, J.E.; Cousens, S.; Mathers, C.; Black, R.E. Global, Regional, and National Causes of Child Mortality in 2000–13, with Projections to Inform Post-2015 Priorities: An Updated Systematic Analysis. *Lancet* **2015**, *385*, 430–440. [CrossRef]
3. Newman, D.E.; Paamoni-Keren, O.; Press, F.; Wiznitzer, A.; Mazor, M.; Sheiner, E. Neonatal outcome in preterm deliveries between 23 and 27 weeks' gestation with and without preterm premature rupture of membranes. *Arch. Gynecol. Obstet.* **2009**, *280*, 7–11. [CrossRef] [PubMed]
4. Jarjour, I.T. Neurodevelopmental outcome after extreme prematurity: A review of the literature. *Pediatr. Neurol.* **2015**, *52*, 143–152. [CrossRef]
5. Lin, C.Y.; Hsu, C.H.; Chang, J.H. Neurodevelopmental outcomes at 2 and 5 years of age in very-low-birth-weight preterm infants born between 2002 and 2009: A prospective cohort study in Taiwan. *Pediatr. Neonatol.* **2020**, *61*, 36–44. [CrossRef]
6. Jameson, R.A.; Bernstein, H.B. Magnesium Sulfate and Novel Therapies to Promote Neuroprotection. *Clin. Perinatol.* **2019**, *46*, 187–201. [CrossRef]
7. Hollanders, J.J.; Schaëfer, N.; Van Der Pal, S.M.; Oosterlaan, J.; Rotteveel, J.; Finken, M.J.J. Long-Term Neurodevelopmental and Functional Outcomes of Infants Born Very Preterm and/or with a Very Low Birth Weight. *Neonatology* **2019**, *115*, 310–319. [CrossRef] [PubMed]
8. Pariente, G.; Wainstock, T.; Walfisch, A.; Landau, D.; Sheiner, E. Placental abruption and long-term neurological hospitalisations in the offspring. *Paediatr. Perinat. Epidemiol.* **2019**, *33*, 215–222. [CrossRef]
9. Bachnas, M.A.; Akbar, M.I.A.; Dachlan, E.G.; Dekker, G. The role of magnesium sulfate (MgSO$_4$) in fetal neuroprotection. *J. Matern. Neonatal. Med.* **2019**, *34*, 966–978. [CrossRef]
10. Hadar, O.; Sheiner, E.; Wainstock, T. The Association Between Delivery of Small-for-Gestational-Age Neonate and Their Risk for Long-Term Neurological Morbidity. *J. Clin. Med.* **2020**, *9*, 3199. [CrossRef]
11. Bashiri, A.; Burstein, E.; Mazor, M. Cerebral palsy and fetal inflammatory response syndrome: A review. *J. Perinat. Med.* **2006**, *34*, 5–12. [CrossRef]
12. Gutvirtz, G.; Wainstock, T.; Masad, R.; Landau, D.; Sheiner, E. Does nuchal cord at birth increase the risk for cerebral palsy? *Early Hum. Dev.* **2019**, *133*, 1–4. [CrossRef]
13. Spittle, A.J.; Morgan, C.; Olsen, J.E.; Novak, I.; Cheong, J.L.Y. Early Diagnosis and Treatment of Cerebral Palsy in Children with a History of Preterm Birth. *Clin. Perinatol.* **2018**, *45*, 409–420. [CrossRef]
14. Hirvonen, M.; Ojala, R.; Korhonen, P.; Haataja, P.; Eriksson, K.; Gissler, M.; Luukkaala, T.; Tammela, O. Cerebral palsy among children born moderately and late preterm. *Pediatrics* **2014**, *134*, e1584–e1593. [CrossRef]
15. Bax, M.; Goldstein, M.; Rosenbaun, P.; Leviton, A.; Paneth, N.; Dan, B.; Jacobsson, B.; Damiano, D. Proposed definition and classification of cerebral palsy, April 2005. *Dev. Med. Child Neurol.* **2005**, *47*, 571–576. [CrossRef] [PubMed]
16. Oskoui, M.; Coutinho, F.; Dykeman, J.; Jetté, N.; Pringsheim, T. An update on the prevalence of cerebral palsy: A systematic review and meta-analysis. *Dev. Med. Child Neurol.* **2013**, *55*, 509–519. [CrossRef]
17. Himpens, E.; Oostra, A.; Franki, I.; Vansteelandt, S.; Vanhaesebrouck, P.; den Broeck, C.V. Predictability of cerebral palsy in a high-risk NICU population. *Early Hum. Dev.* **2010**, *86*, 413–417. [CrossRef]

18. Hagberg, H.; Gressens, P.; Mallard, C. Inflammation during fetal and neonatal life: Implications for neurologic and neuropsychiatric disease in children and adults. *Ann. Neurol.* **2012**, *71*, 444–457. [CrossRef] [PubMed]
19. Fahey, M.C.; Maclennan, A.H.; Kretzschmar, D.; Gecz, J.; Kruer, M.C. The genetic basis of cerebral palsy. *Dev. Med. Child Neurol.* **2017**, *59*, 462–469. [CrossRef]
20. Harding, D.R.; Humphries, S.E.; Whitelaw, A.; Marlow, N.; Montgomery, H.E. Cognitive outcome and cyclo-oxygenase-2 gene (−765 G/C) variation in the preterm infant. *Arch. Dis. Child Fetal. Neonatal Ed.* **2007**, *92*, 108–112. [CrossRef] [PubMed]
21. Casavant, S.G.; Cong, X.; Moore, J.; Starkweather, A. Associations between preterm infant stress, epigenetic alteration, telomere length and neurodevelopmental outcomes: A systematic review. *Early Hum. Dev.* **2019**, *131*, 63–74. [CrossRef]
22. Carlo, W.A.; McDonald, S.A.; Tyson, J.E.; Stoll, B.J.; Ehrenkranz, R.A.; Shankaran, S.; Goldberg, R.N.; Das, A.; Schendel, D.; Thorsen, P.; et al. Cytokines and neurodevelopmental outcomes in extremely low birth weight infants. *J. Pediatr.* **2011**, *159*, 919–925. [CrossRef]
23. Cetral Bureau of Statistics. Population—Statistical Abstract of Israel 2020—No.71. Available online: https://www.cbs.gov.il/en/publications/Pages/2020/Population-Statistical-Abstract-of-Israel-2020-No-71.aspx (accessed on 30 September 2020).
24. Pascal, A.; Govaert, P.; Oostra, A.; Naulaers, G.; Ortibus, E.; Van den Broeck, C. Neurodevelopmental outcome in very preterm and very-low-birthweight infants born over the past decade: A meta-analytic review. *Dev. Med. Child Neurol.* **2018**, *60*, 342–355. [CrossRef]
25. Herber-Jonat, S.; Streiftau, S.; Knauss, E.; Voigt, F.; Flemmer, A.W.; Hummler, H.D.; Schulze, A.; Bode, H. Long-term outcome at age 7–10 years after extreme prematurity-a prospective, two centre cohort study of children born before 25 completed weeks of gestation (1999–2003). *J. Matern. Neonatal. Med.* **2014**, *27*, 1620–1626. [CrossRef]
26. Ream, M.A.; Lehwald, L. Neurologic Consequences of Preterm Birth. *Curr. Neurol. Neurosci. Rep.* **2017**, *18*, 1–10. [CrossRef]
27. Davidesko, S.; Wainstock, T.; Sheiner, E.; Pariente, G. Long-Term Infectious Morbidity of Premature Infants: Is There a Critical Threshold? *J. Clin. Med.* **2020**, *9*, 3008. [CrossRef]
28. Ohana, O.; Wainstock, T.; Sheiner, E.; Leibson, T.; Pariente, G. Long-Term digestive hospitalizations of premature infants (besides necrotizing enterocolitis): Is there a critical threshold? *Arch. Gynecol. Obstet.* **2021**. [CrossRef] [PubMed]
29. Fallang, B.; Hadders-Algra, M. Postural behavior in children born preterm. *Neural Plast.* **2005**, *12*, 175–182. [CrossRef] [PubMed]
30. Ancel, P.Y.; Livinec, F.; Larroque, B.; Marret, S.; Arnaud, C.; Pierrat, V.; Dehan, M.; Sylvie, N.; Escande, B.; Burguet, A.; et al. Cerebral palsy among very preterm children in relation to gestational age and neonatal ultrasound abnormalities: The EPIPAGE cohort study. *Pediatrics* **2006**, *117*, 828–835. [CrossRef] [PubMed]
31. Volpe, J.J. Overview: Normal and abnormal human brain development. *Ment. Retard. Dev. Disabil. Res. Rev.* **2000**, *5*, 1–5. [CrossRef]
32. Lin, G.G.; Scott, J.G. Cytokines and Neurodevelopmental Outcomes in Extremely Low Birth Weight Infants. *J. Pediatr.* **2012**, *100*, 130–134.
33. Andrews, W.W.; Cliver, S.P.; Biasini, F.; Peralta-Carcelen, A.M.; Rector, R.; Alriksson-Schmidt, A.I.; Faye-Petersen, O.; Carlo, W.; Goldenberg, R.; Hauth, J.C. Early preterm birth: Association between in utero exposure to acute inflammation and severe neurodevelopmental disability at 6 years of age. *Am. J. Obstet. Gynecol.* **2008**, *198*, 466.e1. [CrossRef] [PubMed]
34. Cordeiro, C.N.; Tsimis, M.; Burd, I. Infections and brain development. *Obstet. Gynecol. Surv.* **2015**, *70*, 644–655. [CrossRef] [PubMed]

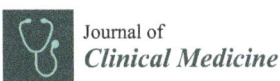

Article

Preterm Delivery; Who Is at Risk?

Dvora Kluwgant [1,†], Tamar Wainstock [2,†], Eyal Sheiner [1,*] and Gali Pariente [1]

[1] Soroka University Medical Center, Department of Obstetrics and Gynecology, Faculty of Health Sciences, Ben-Gurion University of the Negev, Beer-Sheva 8400711, Israel; feinblum@post.bgu.ac.il (D.K.); galipa@bgu.ac.il (G.P.)
[2] School of Public Health, Ben-Gurion University of the Negev, Beer-Sheva 8400711, Israel; wainstoc@bgu.ac.il
* Correspondence: sheiner@bgu.ac.il; Tel.: +972-54-8045074
† The first two authors made an equal contribution.

Abstract: Preterm birth (PTB) is the leading cause of perinatal morbidity and mortality. Adverse effects of preterm birth have a direct correlation with the degree of prematurity, in which infants who are born extremely preterm (24–28 weeks gestation) have the worst outcomes. We sought to determine prominent risk factors for extreme PTB and whether these factors varied between various sub-populations with known risk factors such as previous PTB and multiple gestations. A population-based retrospective cohort study was conducted. Risk factors were examined in cases of extreme PTB in the general population, as well as various sub-groups: singleton and multiple gestations, women with a previous PTB, and women with indicated or induced PTB. A total of 334,415 deliveries were included, of which 1155 (0.35%) were in the extreme PTB group. Placenta previa (OR = 5.8, 95%CI 4.14–8.34, $p < 0.001$), multiple gestations (OR = 7.7, 95% CI 6.58–9.04, $p < 0.001$), and placental abruption (OR = 20.6, 95%CI 17.00–24.96, $p < 0.001$) were the strongest risk factors for extreme PTB. In sub-populations (multiple gestations, women with previous PTB and indicated PTBs), risk factors included placental abruption and previa, lack of prenatal care, and recurrent pregnancy loss. Singleton extreme PTB risk factors included nulliparity, lack of prenatal care, and placental abruption. Placental abruption was the strongest risk factor for extreme preterm birth in all groups, and risk factors did not differ significantly between sub-populations.

Keywords: preterm birth; extreme preterm birth; placental abruption; prematurity

Citation: Kluwgant, D.; Wainstock, T.; Sheiner, E.; Pariente, G. Preterm Delivery; Who Is at Risk?. *J. Clin. Med.* **2021**, *10*, 2279. https://doi.org/10.3390/jcm10112279

Academic Editor: Emmanuel Andrès

Received: 28 April 2021
Accepted: 22 May 2021
Published: 24 May 2021

Publisher's Note: MDPI stays neutral with regard to jurisdictional claims in published maps and institutional affiliations.

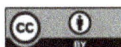

Copyright: © 2021 by the authors. Licensee MDPI, Basel, Switzerland. This article is an open access article distributed under the terms and conditions of the Creative Commons Attribution (CC BY) license (https://creativecommons.org/licenses/by/4.0/).

1. Introduction

Preterm delivery, defined as delivery prior to 37 weeks of gestation, is a leading cause of perinatal morbidity and mortality worldwide, with an incidence of 5–13% depending on location [1]. Since the prevalence of preterm delivery is so high, it is thought to put more financial, medical, and emotional stress on affected communities than any other perinatal issue [2]. Additionally, prematurity has both short and long-standing consequences for affected infants and can leave these individuals with lifelong disabilities, even after the available interventions are attempted [3–5]. Morbidity and mortality are higher among those defined as "very" preterm (<32 weeks) and "extremely" preterm (<28 weeks), but prognosis has improved in recent years with better care, even among those born at 22–23 weeks [6–9]. However, it should be noted that this varies between countries.

Many factors can predispose to the development of preterm delivery, but it is useful to categorize preterm birth into three general etiologic groups: spontaneous labor with intact membranes, preterm premature rupture of membranes (PPROM) leading to preterm delivery, and labor induction due to maternal or fetal factors [4,10]. These categories each have their own common risk factors; for example, risk factors for PPROM-induced delivery include intrauterine infection [11], tobacco use [12], abruption [13], multiple gestations [14], previous PPROM [15], and cervical factors [16,17], among others. However, these risk factors are not exclusive to each etiologic group, and some can be risk factors for multiple groups.

Other risk factors include previous C section [18], low pre-pregnancy BMI [19], and hypertensive disorders of pregnancy [20]. Women who have had one previous spontaneous preterm delivery have an increased risk of subsequent preterm delivery in their next pregnancy, with an absolute risk of about 30% of another preterm delivery [21,22]. Primigravid women and those carrying male fetuses also have a higher association with preterm delivery [2]. Even seemingly insignificant factors such as ambient air temperature can have an impact on rates of preterm delivery [23].

While various risk factors for preterm delivery are well recognized, it is still unclear whether the cause of preterm delivery is multifactorial, or whether each risk factor leads to a different pathophysiologic cause of preterm delivery [1]. In this study, we attempt to evaluate the impact of different known risk factors on the occurrence of extremely preterm birth (<28 weeks) while controlling for confounders. We also examine whether different risk factors for preterm delivery were more important in various subgroups, such as induced versus spontaneous preterm birth and multiple versus singleton gestations.

2. Materials and Methods

2.1. Population and Study Design

This retrospective cohort study was performed using data from the birthing center at Soroka University Medical Center (SUMC). SUMC is the largest tertiary hospital in the Negev region of Israel and serves the entire population of this area. Data were collected using the computerized perinatal database. Information from the perinatal database is first documented directly following delivery by an attending physician. Subsequently, medical secretaries routinely review the information before it is entered into the database. After evaluating prenatal care records together with the routine hospital documents, coding is performed. These measures ensure maximal completeness and accurateness of the databases. The databases include demographic information and International Classification of Diseases, 9th revision codes (ICD-9) for all diagnoses. The institutional review board, in accordance with the Helsinki declaration, approved the study (0358-19-SOR). All deliveries between the years 1991 and 2018 were included. Cases of fetal malformations or chromosomal abnormalities of the fetus were excluded from the study.

Four groups were examined based on gestational age, as put forth by the WHO: extreme preterm (24 + 0–27 + 6 weeks), very preterm (28 + 1–31 + 6 weeks), and moderate to late preterm (32 + 0–36 + 6 weeks), with a reference group of term births (>37 + 0 weeks) [24]. We examined the following obstetric risk factors and evaluated their impact on the occurrence of preterm birth in different gestational ages while controlling for confounders: maternal age, ethnicity, nulliparity, previous cesarean delivery, recurrent pregnancy loss, diabetes mellitus, hypertension, use of in vitro fertilization or ovarian induction, lack of prenatal care, gestational diabetes mellitus, preeclampsia, placenta previa, placental abruption, as well as delivery characteristics such as cesarean delivery, assisted delivery, maternal need for blood transfusions after delivery, post-partum hemorrhage, and fetal characteristics such as fetal gender, small for gestational age fetus, 5-min APGAR score <7, umbilical cord pH <7, intrapartum death, and number of fetuses. Placental abruption was clinically defined as the premature detachment of an implanted placenta from the uterine wall before the delivery of the fetus. The diagnosis was made by the attending staff during the delivery [25,26]. In some of the cases, the diagnosis was confirmed by pathological examination. Nevertheless, as abruption is considered a clinical diagnosis, only some cases of acute abruptions demonstrated histologic confirmation. Maternal exposure, with or without placenta abruption, as well as all other clinical characteristics were identified using ICD-9 codes, with ICD-9 code 641.2 for placental abruption. Placenta previa occurs when the placenta attaches inside the uterus but in an abnormal position near or over the cervical opening [27]. As the diagnosis of placenta previa may change later in pregnancy, we defined it here as placenta previa diagnosed on ultrasound before delivery during routine ultrasounds, which in Israel are performed at 14, 22, and 30 weeks, and also every time a woman presents for prenatal care.

We further examined whether different risk factors and outcomes for preterm delivery were more important in various subgroups; induced vs. spontaneous preterm birth, those with vs. without previous PTB, and multiples vs. singletons. The vast majority of multiples born at our center were twins (65.5%), with the remainder being triplets (6.6%) or quadruplets (0.7%). Therefore, we did not differentiate between twins and higher order multiples, since the rates of higher order multiples were exceedingly low (twins = 3.4%, triplets = 0.1%).

2.2. Statistical Analysis

Statistical analysis was performed using SPSS (SPSS, Chicago, IL, USA). We used the Chi-square test to calculate the statistical significance based on differences between qualitative variables and the *t* for continuous variables. Few multivariable logistic regression models were created in order to examine independent risk factors for preterm delivery according to gestational age and among different sub-groups, while controlling for confounders. Odds ratios and their 95% confidence intervals were calculated, and *p*-values less than 0.05 were considered statistically significant.

3. Results

A total of 334,415 births were included in our study, including extreme PTB (n = 1155), very PTB (n = 2490), moderate-late PTB (n = 25,344), and term births (n = 304,732). Characteristics of the overall population are summarized in Table 1. There was a significantly higher rate of PTB in Bedouin women, especially in the very PTB group (57.1%, $p < 0.001$). The rate of nulliparity was significantly higher in the extreme PTB group (37.3%, $p < 0.001$). Rates of recurrent pregnancy loss, lack of prenatal care, placenta previa and abruption, need for maternal blood transfusion, postpartum hemorrhage, small for gestational age neonates, 5-min APGAR score <7, umbilical cord pH <7, and intrapartum death were also all significantly higher in the extreme PTB group than in all others. Those in the very preterm group had the highest rates of hypertension, use of in vitro fertilization and ovulation induction, preeclampsia, delivery by cesarean delivery, multiple gestations, and male fetal gender. Rates of previous cesarean delivery were 25.7%, 27.9%, 25.9%, and 15.3% for extreme PTB, very PTB, moderate–late PTB, and term deliveries, respectively $p < 0.001$. Rates of previous PTB were 27.5%, 30.1%, 28.8%, and 11.1% for extreme PTB, very PTB, moderate–late PTB, and term deliveries, respectively $p < 0.001$. Rates of small for gestational age infants were 14.2%, 6.2%, 4.3%, and 4.7% among extreme PTB, very PTB, moderate PTB, and term deliveries, respectively, $p < 0.001$. Rates of large for gestational age infants were 0.1%, 0.2%, 0.4%, and 4.8% among extreme PTB, very PTB, moderate PTB, and term deliveries, respectively, $p < 0.001$. Finally, those in the moderate–late PTB group had the highest rates of diabetes mellitus and gestational diabetes mellitus, while the term births had the highest percentage of Jewish mothers and female neonates.

Logistic regression (Table 2) showed placental abruption to be the most significant independent risk factor in the extreme PTB group (OR = 13.579, CI = 8.757–21.057, $p < 0.001$). Other factors that were independent risk factors in this gestational age group were lack of prenatal care, nulliparity, placenta previa, recurrent pregnancy loss, induction of labor, and multiple gestation. In the other PTB groups (Table 3), abruption was also the most significant risk factor (OR = 22.799, CI = 18.422–28.216, $p < 0.001$). Interestingly, having a history of diabetes mellitus (OR = 0.362, CI = 0.238–0.552, $p < 0.001$) decreased the probability of PTB in this gestational age group. Adding the child's year of birth to the logistic regression model did not significantly affect the results of the model. The only variable that lost its significance as risk factor for extreme PTB was preeclampsia.

Table 1. Characteristics of general population.

Characteristic:	Extreme PTB: 24 + 0–27 + 6 Weeks	Very PTB: 28 + 1–31 + 6 Weeks	Moderate–Late PTB: 32 + 0- 36 + 6 Weeks	Term Birth: >37 + 0 weeks	p-Value *	p-Value **
n	1155	2490	25,344	304,732		
Maternal Age (mean ± SD)	28.07 ± 6.642	28.32 ± 6.362	28.40 ± 6.186	28.19 ± 5.798	0.176	0.499
Ethnicity: Jewish	46.7	42.9	48.1	48.4	<0.001	0.268
Bedouin	53.3	57.1	51.9	51.6		
Nulliparity	37.3	31.9	29.7	23.8	<0.001	<0.001
Previous PTB ***	27.5	30.1	28.8	11.1	<0.001	<0.001
Previous cesarean delivery	25.7	27.9	25.9	15.3	<0.001	<0.001
Recurrent pregnancy loss	8.7	7.8	6.6	4.6	<0.001	<0.001
Diabetes mellitus	2.3	6.1	7.9	5.1	<0.001	<0.001
Hypertension	9.1	14.8	12.2	4.4	<0.001	<0.001
In vitro fertilization	7.2	8.6	6.4	1.3	<0.001	<0.001
Ovulation induction	2.9	4.7	3.5	0.9		
Lack of prenatal care	13.5	12.4	8.4	9.0	<0.001	<0.001
Gestational diabetes mellitus	1.2	4.1	5.4	4.0	<0.001	<0.001
Preeclampsia	7	13.6	10.5	3.5	<0.001	<0.001
Placenta previa	3.6	3.3	2.1	0.2	<0.001	<0.001
Placental abruption	12.8	10.2	2.4	0.3	<0.001	<0.001
Cesarean delivery	16.1	19.1	18.2	11.7	<0.001	<0.001
Assisted delivery	0.2	0.5	1.6	3.3	<0.001	<0.001
Blood transfusion	7.8	6.5	3.6	1.3	<0.001	<0.001
Postpartum hemorrhage	1.0	0.5	0.4	0.6	<0.001	0.030
Multiple gestation	22.1	26.9	23.2	1.6	<0.001	<0.001
Neonate's Gender: Male	53.0	53.1	52.4	50.8	<0.001	0.164
Female	47.0	46.9	47.6	49.2		
Small for gestational age neonate	14.2	6.2	4.3	4.7	<0.001	<0.001
5-min APGAR < 7	28.6	6.4	1.3	0.3	<0.001	<0.001
Umbilical Cord pH < 7	2.9	0.9	0.9	0.4	0.007	0.026
Intrapartum death	5.0	0.6	0.1	0.0	<0.001	<0.001

* p-value for multiple comparisons (all four groups); ** p-value for comparison between the extreme PTB and all other groups; *** This analysis was restricted to women with birth order >1. APGAR: The APGAR score (named after Dr. Virginia Apgar) is a universal scoring system use to assess newborns one minute and five minutes after they are born.

Table 2. Logistic regression results for extreme preterm group.

Characteristic	Adjusted Odds Ratio	95% Confidence Interval	Significance (p-Value)
Lack of prenatal care	2.019	1.694–2.407	<0.001
In vitro fertilization	1.338	1.038–1.723	0.024
Nulliparity	2.304	2.006–2.647	0.071
Previous cesarean delivery	1.444	1.212–1.720	<0.001
Diabetes mellitus	0.322	0.217–0.477	<0.001
Preeclampsia	1.033	0.816–1.307	<0.001
Placenta previa	5.884	4.149–8.344	<0.001
Recurrent pregnancy loss	1.815	1.468–2.245	<0.001
Placental abruption	20.606	17.006–24.969	<0.001
Induction of labor	1.410	1.220–1.626	<0.001
Multiple gestation	7.714	6.581–9.042	<0.001

Table 3. Risk factors in women with previous PTB.

Characteristic:	Extreme PTB: 24 + 0–27 + 6 Weeks	Very PTB: 28 + 1–31 + 6 Weeks	Moderate–Late PTB: 32 + 0–36 + 6 Weeks	Term Birth: >37 + 0 weeks	p-Value *	p-Value **
n	204	514	5173	26,046	–	
Ethnicity: Bedouin	64.7	62.8	58.1	63.5	<0.001	0.537
Jewish	35.3	37.6	41.9	36.5		
Previous cesarean delivery	31.9	40.3	36.9	29.0	<0.001	0.661
Diabetes mellitus	1.5	6.6	9.1	6.7	<0.001	0.002
Hypertension	12.7	17.9	12.3	5.3	<0.001	0.001
In vitro fertilization	4.4	4.7	3.7	1.3	<0.001	0.005
Ovulation induction	1.5	3.1	1.5	0.5		
Gestational diabetes mellitus	1.5	4.1	5.7	5.0	<0.001	0.018
Preeclampsia	11.3	15.4	9.5	3.6	<0.001	<0.001
Placenta previa	4.4	3.5	1.8	0.3	<0.001	<0.001
Placental abruption	14.2	11.5	2.8	0.4	<0.001	<0.001

* p-value for multiple comparisons (all four groups); ** p-value for comparison between the extreme PTB and all other group.

In the extreme PTB group (Table 3), those who had a history of previous PTB had the highest rates of Bedouin ethnicity, placenta previa, need for maternal blood transfusion, postpartum hemorrhage, female fetal gender, small for gestational age neonates, and 5-min APGAR <7. The other PTB groups in those with a history of PTB, the highest rates of previous cesarean delivery, diabetes mellitus, hypertension, use of in vitro fertilization and ovulation induction, gestational diabetes mellitus, preeclampsia, cesarean delivery, male neonatal gender, and intrapartum death were seen. Notably, term babies born to women both with and without a history of PTB had the highest rates of assisted delivery. Similar to those in the general population, placental abruption was the highest risk factor for PTB (OR = 13.579, CI = 8.757–21.057, p = 0.001) in this population according to multivariate analysis (Table 4). Placental abruption was found to be more common among pregnancies with preeclampsia compared to pregnancies without preeclampsia (1.7% vs. 0.5%, OR 3.3, 95% CI 2.93–3.86, p < 0.001). A positive non-parametric correlation was demonstrated between the two variables, even though the correlation was very weak.

Table 4. Logistic regression results for women with previous PTB.

Characteristic	Adjusted Odds Ratio	95% Confidence Interval	Significance (p-Value)
Lack of prenatal care	2.174	1.391–3.399	0.001
In vitro fertilization	1.358	0.659–2.797	0.407
Previous cesarean delivery	1.013	0.746–1.378	0.932
Diabetes mellitus	0.162	0.051–0.510	0.002
Preeclampsia	1.888	1.193–2.991	0.007
Placenta previa	4.161	1.958–8.839	<0.001
Recurrent pregnancy loss	2.370	1.664–3.374	<0.001
Placental abruption	13.579	8.757–21.057	<0.001
Induction of labor	1.478	1.018–2.145	0.040
Multiple gestation	6.177	4.202–9.080	<0.001

In singleton deliveries, the rates of nulliparity (Table 5), history of recurrent pregnancy loss, use of in vitro fertilization, lack of prenatal care, placenta previa, abruption, need for maternal blood transfusion, postpartum hemorrhage, small for gestational age neonate, 5-min APGAR <7, and intrapartum death were all highest in the extreme PTB group. For the other PTB groups, there were higher rates of Bedouin ethnicity, previous PTB and cesarean delivery, diabetes mellitus, hypertension, use of ovulation induction, gestational diabetes mellitus, preeclampsia, cesarean delivery, and assisted delivery.

Table 5. Risk factors for singleton pregnancies.

Characteristic:	Extreme PTB: 24 + 0–27 + 6 Weeks	Very PTB: 28 + 1–31 + 6 Weeks	Moderate–Late PTB: 32 + 0–36 + 6 Weeks	Term Birth: >37 + 0 Weeks	p-Value *	p-Value **
n	905	1829	19,508	299,814	-	
Ethnicity: Bedouin	53.3	58.0	53.9	51.7	<0.001	0.386
Jewish	46.7	42.0	46.1	48.3		
Nulliparity	35.4	29.1	28.9	23.8	<0.001	<0.001
Previous PTB	18.4	22.1	22.9	8.6	<0.001	
Previous cesarean delivery	17.6	19.5	19.5	11.7	<0.001	<0.001
Recurrent pregnancy loss	8.4	8.0	6.7	4.6	<0.001	<0.001
Diabetes mellitus	2.1	4.8	7.4	5.0	<0.001	<0.001
Hypertension	10.3	17.1	12.0	4.3	<0.001	<0.001
In vitro fertilization	2.6	2.3	2.1	1.1	<0.001	<0.001
Ovulation induction	1.0	1.4	1.1	0.8		
Lack of prenatal care	15.6	13.7	9.7	9.0	<0.001	<0.001
Gestational diabetes mellitus	1.0	3.2	4.9	4.0	<0.001	<0.001
Preeclampsia	8.2	15.8	10.2	3.4	<0.001	<0.001
Placenta Previa	4.1	4.1	2.5	0.2	<0.001	<0.001

* p-value for multiple comparisons (all four groups); ** p-value for comparison between the extreme PTB and all other groups.

According to logistic regression (Table 6), the greatest risk factor for PTB in this group was placental abruption (OR = 24.619, CI = 20.063–30.210, $p < 0.001$).

Table 6. Logistic regression results for singleton gestation group.

Characteristic	Adjusted Odds Ratio	95% Confidence Interval	Significance
Lack of prenatal care	2.136	1.772–2.574	<0.001
In vitro fertilization	1.687	1.104–2.580	0.016
Nulliparity	2.226	1.902–2.605	<0.001
Previous cesarean delivery	1.592	1.314–1.929	<0.001
Diabetes mellitus	0.345	0.218–0.545	<0.001
Preeclampsia	1.432	1.117–1.837	0.005
Placenta previa	5.845	4.022–8.945	<0.001
Recurrent pregnancy loss	1.747	1.368–2.232	<0.001
Placental abruption	24.619	20.063–30.210	<0.001
Previous PTB	2.305	1.980–2.784	<0.001
Induction of labor	1.528	1.312–1.778	<0.001

In multiple gestations (Table 7), rates of nulliparity, placenta previa, placental abruption, need for maternal blood transfusion, small for gestational age neonate, 5-min APGAR < 7, and intrapartum death were highest in the extreme PTB group. The other PTB groups had the highest rates of Bedouin ethnicity, previous PTB and cesarean delivery, diabetes mellitus, hypertension, use of in vitro fertilization or ovulation induction, lack of prenatal care, gestational diabetes mellitus, preeclampsia, cesarean delivery, male neonatal gender, and umbilical cord pH > 7. Term babies in both single and multiple gestations had the highest rates of assisted deliveries. In the logistic regression (Table 8), placental abruption was the most significant risk factor for extreme PTB in multiple gestations (OR = 7.467, CI = 4.398–12.677, p < 0.001). Those with diabetes mellitus and preeclampsia had a negative risk for extreme PTB (OR = 0.280, CI = 0.131–0.598, p = 0.001; OR = −0.229, CI = 1.779 = 12.819, p < 0.001, respectively). We did not differentiate between twins and higher-order multiples, since the rates of higher-order multiples were exceedingly low (twins = 3.4%, triplets = 0.1%).

Table 7. Risk factors for multiple gestations.

Characteristic:	Extreme PTB: 24 + 0–27 + 6 Weeks	Very PTB: 28 + 1–31 + 6 Weeks	Moderate–Late PTB: 32 + 0–36 + 6 Weeks	Term Birth: >37 + 0 Weeks	p-Value *	p-Value **
n	255	670	5888	4960	–	
Ethnicity: Bedouin	53.3	54.6	45.1	47.1	<0.001	0.031
Jewish	46.7	45.4	54.9	52.9		
Nulliparity	43.9	39.4	32.5	24.3	<0.001	<0.001
Previous PTB	14.9	16.6	12.3	7.1	<0.001	
Previous cesarean delivery	11.0	18.1	13.9	10.4	<0.001	0.436
Recurrent pregnancy loss	9.8	7.3	6.3	6.1	0.084	0.023
Diabetes mellitus	2.7	9.7	9.4	8.4	<0.001	<0.001
Hypertension	4.7	8.5	12.9	8.3	<0.001	0.002
In vitro fertilization	23.5	25.7	20.4	14.9	<0.001	0.106
Ovulation induction	9.4	13.9	11.6	8.9		
Lack of prenatal care	6.3	9.0	4.1	5.3	<0.001	0.308
Gestational diabetes mellitus	2.0	6.7	7.3	6.9	0.013	0.002
Preeclampsia	2.7	7.6	11.6	7.2	<0.001	<0.001
Placenta Previa	2.0	0.9	0.5	0.2	<0.001	<0.001
Placental Abruption	7.1	4.5	0.9	0.7	<0.001	<0.001

* p-value for multiple comparisons (all four groups); ** p-value for comparison between the extreme PTB and all other groups.

Table 8. Logistic regression results for multiple gestation group.

Characteristic	Adjusted Odds Ratio	95% Confidence Interval	Significance
Lack of prenatal care	1.396	0.823–2.368	0.216
In vitro fertilization	1.171	0.856–1.604	0.324
Nulliparity	2.483	1.855–3.323	<0.001
Previous cesarean delivery	0.909	0.589–1.401	0.664
Diabetes mellitus	0.280	0.131–0.598	0.001
Preeclampsia	0.229	0.107–0.490	<0.001
Placenta previa	4.775	1.779–12.819	0.002
Recurrent pregnancy loss	1.853	1.207–2.846	0.005
Placental abruption	7.467	4.398–12.677	<0.001
Previous PTB	2.113	1.435–3.112	<0.001
Induction of Labor	0.424	0.198–0.907	0.027

In those with induced PTB (Table 9), higher rates of Jewish ethnicity, recurrent pregnancy loss, use of in vitro fertilization, placenta previa, need for maternal blood transfusion, postpartum hemorrhage, small for gestational age neonate, 5-min APGAR < 7, and intrapartum death were seen in the extreme PTB group. In the other induced PTB groups, higher rates of previous PTB and cesarean delivery, diabetes mellitus, hypertension, use of ovulation induction, lack of prenatal care, preeclampsia, cesarean delivery, maternal blood transfusion, and multiple gestations were seen. In the logistic regression (Table 10), the most important risk factor for induced extreme PTB was abruption (OR = 14.175, CI = 8.654–23.218, $p < 0.001$). Diabetes mellitus had a negative predictive value for induced extreme PTD (OR = 0.262, CI = 0.123–0.556, $p < 0.001$). Adding child's year of birth to the logistic regression models of other sub-populations (previous PTB, singleton pregnancies, multiple gestations and indicated PTBs) did not affect significantly the results of the models.

Table 9. Risk factors for Induced PTB.

Characteristic:	Extreme PTB: 24 + 0–27 + 6 Weeks	Very PTB: 28 + 1–31 + 6 Weeks	Moderate–Late PTB: 32 + 0- 36 + 6 Weeks	Term Birth: >37 + 0 Weeks	p-Value *	p-Value **
n	281	346	4153	70,615		
Ethnicity: Bedouin	44.8	55.2	42.7	38.5	<0.001	0.083
Jewish	55.2	44.8	57.3	61.5		
Nulliparity	40.6	32.7	42.0	39.4	<0.001	0.719
Previous PTB	13.5	16.2	17.4	6.2	<0.001	
Previous cesarean delivery	10.0	11.3	5.3	4.6	<0.001	<0.001
Recurrent pregnancy loss	7.8	7.5	6.6	4.8	<0.001	0.023
Diabetes mellitus	2.5	5.2	8.6	9.0	<0.001	<0.001
Hypertension	11.7	14.7	24.3	9.0	<0.001	0.313
In vitro fertilization	2.5	2.0	3.0	1.8	<0.001	0.672
Ovulation induction	1.8	2.0	2.3	1.4		
Lack of prenatal care	11.7	12.4	5.7	4.8	<0.001	<0.001
Gestational diabetes mellitus	1.4	3.2	5.8	6.9	<0.001	<0.001
Preeclampsia	8.9	13.9	21.3	7.5	<0.001	0.716
Placenta previa	1.4	0.3	0.2	0.1	<0.001	<0.001
Placental Abruption	7.1	7.2	1.8	0.3	<0.001	<0.001

* p-value for multiple comparisons (all four groups); ** p-value for comparison between the extreme PTB and all other groups.

Table 10. Logistic regression results for Induced PTB group.

Characteristic	Adjusted Odds Ratio	95% Confidence Interval	Significance
Lack of prenatal care	2.585	1.771–3.713	<0.001
In vitro fertilization	1.205	0.557–2.608	0.635
Nulliparity	1.331	1.024–1.729	0.032
Previous cesarean delivery	2.177	1.430–3.315	<0.001
Diabetes mellitus	0.262	0.123–0.556	<0.001
Preeclampsia	0.954	0.628–1.449	0.825
Placenta previa	9.193	2.867–29.484	<0.001
Recurrent pregnancy loss	1.611	1.030–2.521	0.037
Placental abruption	14.175	8.654–23.218	<0.001
History of PTD	2.013	1.383–2.292	<0.001

4. Discussion

The results of our study add to the growing body of information on this topic and provide data specific to the population under study, leaving room for further investigation. In this study, the most notable outcome we found was that placental abruption (defined here as clinically diagnosed placental abruption) was the risk factor with the highest significance in all of the populations and sub-populations (e.g., early PTB multiples, induced early PTB, etc.) that we looked at. As placental abruption is a clinical diagnosis, its association with induction of labor may be due to the clinical decision to induce labor following a suspected abruption or may be related to abruption caused by the induction itself. Another interesting finding of our study is that in our population, having diabetes mellitus had an inverse relationship with risk of early PTB. Preeclampsia also showed a weak, negatively predictive effect on extreme PTB, but this was non-statistically significant. Rates of assisted delivery (which at our facility entails use of vacuum extraction) were lower than in other settings as well; these rates are indeed low, since in our medical center, vacuum is hardly performed in preterm deliveries [28].

As is well known and widely noted in other studies, placental abruption is often associated with preterm delivery [10,13]. This risk factor is very significant, with the risk being estimated as between 1.2 and 31.7, and incidence being between 40 and 60% [13]. Placental abruption has been shown by other studies to be nine times more likely to occur in preterm gestational ages than is in term gestational ages (2.8% versus 0.3%, respectively) [29]. Still, other studies have shown that placental abruption implicates itself in 5.8% of births occurring before 35 weeks of gestation, with another finding that 50% of women with PTB had "clinical or histological abruption, chorioamnionitis, or both" [30,31].

Placental abruption is defined as a premature detachment of the placenta from the uterine wall, which occurs after 20 weeks of gestation but before birth. Typical presenting will include vaginal bleeding, abdominal pain, contractions, and abnormal fetal heart rate tracings. Placental abruption leads to uteroplacental under perfusion, hypoxia, and placental ischemia. Thus, abruption can cause a spontaneous PTB, but it may also be an indication for an induced PTB in order to save the life of the mother or her fetus. The mechanism by which placental abruption causes spontaneous PTB is believed to be due to blood irritating the uterine lining and stimulating contractions, which may subsequently lead to PTB [13].

There are a few reasons why placental abruption was found to be the most significant risk factor for PTB in our study. Firstly, abruption was found to have the highest incidence during weeks 24–26 [32], which is a timeframe that falls into the early PTB gestational age group, explaining the high odds ratio seen with abruption in this group. Additionally, over 50% of abruption occurs before term, meaning that if abruption occurs and leads to a natural or induced delivery, it is highly likely that the neonate will be premature. One area our study did not explore was whether the rates of women with risk factors (such as smoking, use of cocaine, etc.) for abruption had a higher rate of PTB caused by abruption, this is an area that is ripe for exploration, as it may help explain our results.

Many studies show that gestational diabetes mellitus and pregestational diabetes mellitus can lead to an increased risk of preterm birth. This being said, there is no consensus as to whether diabetes mellitus is an independent risk factor for spontaneous PTB. Some studies have demonstrated an increased risk of PTB in both pregestational and gestational diabetes [33], while others indicated that this risk was associated only with insulin-treated diabetes mellitus [34]. One study showed obesity to have protective effects against preterm birth [35], which could help explain the results seen in our population, as women with diabetes mellitus are more likely to be obese.

The uncertainty of the effect of gestational diabetes mellitus in our study may be related to the fact that instead of categorizing diabetes mellitus as gestational versus pregestational, we used a composite outcome that included all cases of diabetes mellitus in pregnancy. Since the mechanism of placental pathology is likely different in these two entities, more clear results may be obtained by studying these as separate pathologies and looking at the effect of each on the risk of PTB.

The strengths of this study lie in the fact that it was performed using a very large perinatal database with many years of delivery information about mothers and their neonates. This gave us access to a large population from which we could aggregate data and determine the results. Another strength of this study was that we used sub-group analysis, which allowed us to examine each risk factor on its own while controlling for confounders. The most significant limitation to this study is that it was done retrospectively, and therefore, the results do not indicate causation but rather correlation between the risk factors and outcomes. Another weakness lies in the fact that we did not have data to perform distinct analyses on the risks of extreme PTB in monochorionic versus dichorionic twins and rather regarded them as one entity ('multiple gestations'). Additionally, the rate of extreme PBT in our population was significantly lower than that of other populations. It should be noted that some populations report lower rates of extreme PTB; this may be due to differences among populations [36]. Since our study focused on gestational age, we did not perform any analyses based on birthweight centile. This may have added to the completeness of our data. Overall, however, since we were able to use a large population with a long follow up and had significant results, this study is still able to shed light on the topic at hand.

5. Conclusions

Our study suggested a strong association between early PTB and placental abruption. Since the most significant risk factor for placental abruption is a previous placental abruption, a future area for research may be looking at rates of early PTB due to abruption in those with previous placental abruption. Another interesting feature of placental abruption is that the risk factors for abruption differ in term versus preterm abruption, but the exact difference in mechanism is not well understood, leaving this area open to further investigation.

Author Contributions: Conceptualization, D.K., E.S. and G.P.; methodology T.W.; software, T.W.; validation, T.W.; formal analysis, D.K.; investigation, D.K.; resources, G.P.; data curation, T.W.; writing—original draft preparation, D.K.; writing—review and editing, D.K., G.P. and E.S.; visualization, D.K.; supervision, G.P.; project diabetes mellitus administration, G.P. All authors have read and agreed to the published version of the manuscript.

Funding: This research received no external funding.

Institutional Review Board Statement: The study was conducted according to the guidelines of the Declaration of Helsinki, and approved by the Institutional Review Board (or Ethics Committee) of Ben Gurion University of the Negev.

Informed Consent Statement: Due to the retrospective nature of the study and the use of previously obtained computerized data, patient consent was not sought.

Data Availability Statement: The data presented in this study are available on request from the corresponding author. The data are not publicly available due to restrictions e.g., privacy or ethical.

Conflicts of Interest: The authors declare no conflict of interest.

References

1. Jiang, M.; Mishu, M.M.; Lu, D.; Yin, X. A case control study of risk factors and neonatal outcomes of preterm birth. *Taiwan J. Obstet. Gynecol.* **2018**, *57*, 814–818. [CrossRef] [PubMed]
2. Martin, J.N., Jr.; D'Alton, M.; Jacobsson, B.; Norman, J.E. In Pursuit of Progress Toward Effective Preterm Birth Reduction. *Obstet. Gynecol.* **2017**, *129*, 715–719. [CrossRef] [PubMed]
3. Murray, S.R.; Stock, S.J.; Norman, J.E. Long-term childhood outcomes after interventions for prevention and management of preterm birth. *Semin. Perinatol.* **2017**, *41*, 519–527. [CrossRef] [PubMed]
4. Simmons, L.E.; Rubens, C.E.; Darmstadt, G.L.; Gravett, M.G. Preventing preterm birth and neonatal mortality: Exploring the epidemiology, causes, and interventions. *Semin. Perinatol.* **2010**, *34*, 408–415. [CrossRef]
5. Padeh, E.; Wainstock, T.; Sheiner, E.; Landau, D.; Walfisch, A. Gestational age and the long-term impact on children's infectious urinary morbidity. *Arch. Gynecol. Obstet.* **2019**, *299*, 385–392. [CrossRef]
6. Kusuda, S.; Fujimura, M.; Sakuma, I.; Aotani, H.; Kabe, K.; Itani, Y.; Ichiba, H.; Matsunami, K.; Nishida, H. Morbidity and mortality of infants with very low birth weight in Japan: Center variation. *Pediatrics* **2006**, *118*, e1130–e1138. [CrossRef]
7. Norman, M.; Hallberg, B.; Abrahamsson, T.; Björklund, L.J.; Domellöf, M.; Farooqi, A.; Foyn Bruun, C.; Gadsbøll, C.; Hellström-Westas, L.; Ingemansson, F.; et al. Association Between Year of Birth and 1-Year Survival Among Extremely Preterm Infants in Sweden During 2004–2007 and 2014–2016. *JAMA* **2019**, *321*, 1188–1199. [CrossRef]
8. Mehler, K.; Oberthuer, A.; Keller, T.; Becker, I.; Valter, M.; Roth, B.; Kribs, A. Survival Among Infants Born at 22 or 23 Weeks' Gestation Following Active Prenatal and Postnatal Care. *JAMA Pediatr.* **2016**, *170*, 671–677. [CrossRef]
9. Watkins, P.L.; Dagle, J.M.; Bell, E.F.; Colaizy, T.T. Outcomes at 18 to 22 Months of Corrected Age for Infants Born at 22 to 25 Weeks of Gestation in a Center Practicing Active Management. *J. Pediatr.* **2020**, *217*, 52–58.e1. [CrossRef]
10. Goldenberg, R.L.; Culhane, J.F.; Iams, J.D.; Romero, R. Epidemiology and causes of preterm birth. *Lancet* **2008**, *371*, 75–84. [CrossRef]
11. Goldenberg, R.L.; Hauth, J.C.; Andrews, W.W. Intrauterine infection and preterm delivery. *N. Engl. J. Med.* **2000**, *342*, 1500–1507. [CrossRef]
12. Dahlin, S.; Gunnerbeck, A.; Wikstrom, A.K.; Cnattingius, S.; Edstedt Bonamy, A.K. Maternal tobacco use and extremely premature birth—A population-based cohort study. *BJOG Int. J. Obstet. Gynaecol.* **2016**, *123*, 1938–1946. [CrossRef]
13. Downes, K.L.; Grantz, K.L.; Shenassa, E.D. Maternal, Labor, Delivery, and Perinatal Outcomes Associated with Placental Abruption: A Systematic Review. *Am. J. Perinatol.* **2017**, *34*, 935–957. [CrossRef]
14. Fuchs, F.; Senat, M.V. Multiple gestations and preterm birth. *Semin. Fetal Neonatal Med.* **2016**, *21*, 113–120. [CrossRef]
15. Lee, T.; Carpenter, M.W.; Heber, W.W.; Silver, H.M. Preterm premature rupture of membranes: Risks of recurrent complications in the next pregnancy among a population-based sample of gravid women. *Am. J. Obstet. Gynecol.* **2003**, *188*, 209–213. [CrossRef]
16. Iams, J.D.; Goldenberg, R.L.; Meis, P.J.; Mercer, B.M.; Moawad, A.; Das, A.; Thom, E.; McNellis, D.; Copper, R.L.; Johnson, F.; et al. The length of the cervix and the risk of spontaneous premature delivery. National Institute of Child Health and Human Development Maternal Fetal Medicine Unit Network. *N. Engl. J. Med.* **1996**, *334*, 567–572. [CrossRef]
17. Hamou, B.; Sheiner, E.; Coreanu, T.; Walfisch, A.; Silberstein, T. Intrapartum cervical lacerations and their impact on future pregnancy outcome. *J. Matern. Fetal Neonatal Med.* **2018**, *33*, 883–887. [CrossRef]
18. Williams, C.M.; Asaolu, I.; Chavan, N.R.; Williamson, L.H.; Lewis, A.M.; Beaven, L.; Ashford, K.B. Previous cesarean delivery associated with subsequent preterm birth in the United States. *Eur. J. Obstet. Gynecol. Reprod. Biol.* **2018**, *229*, 88–93. [CrossRef]
19. Lengyel, C.S.; Ehrlich, S.; Iams, J.D.; Muglia, L.J.; DeFranco, E.A. Effect of Modifiable Risk Factors on Preterm Birth: A Population Based-Cohort. *Matern. Child Health J.* **2017**, *21*, 777–785. [CrossRef]
20. Davies, E.L.; Bell, J.S.; Bhattacharya, S. Preeclampsia and preterm delivery: A population-based case-control study. *Hypertens. Pregnancy* **2016**, *35*, 510–519. [CrossRef]
21. Phillips, C.; Velji, Z.; Hanly, C.; Metcalfe, A. Risk of recurrent spontaneous preterm birth: A systematic review and meta-analysis. *BMJ Open* **2017**, *7*, e015402. [CrossRef] [PubMed]
22. Grantz, K.L.; Hinkle, S.N.; Mendola, P.; Sjaarda, L.A.; Leishear, K.; Albert, P.S. Differences in risk factors for recurrent versus incident preterm delivery. *Am. J. Epidemiol.* **2015**, *182*, 157–167. [CrossRef] [PubMed]
23. Walfisch, A.; Kabakov, E.; Friger, M.; Sheiner, E. Trends, seasonality and effect of ambient temperature on preterm delivery. *J. Matern. Fetal Neonatal Med.* **2017**, *30*, 2483–2487. [CrossRef] [PubMed]
24. World Health Organization. Preterm Birth. 2018. Available online: https://www.who.int/en/news-room/fact-sheets/detail/preterm-birth (accessed on 1 January 2021).
25. Pariente, G.; Wainstock, T.; Walfisch, A.; Landau, D.; Sheiner, E. Placental abruption and long-term neurological hospitalisations in the offspring. *Paediatr. Perinat. Epidemiol.* **2019**, *33*, 215–222. [CrossRef]
26. Pariente, G.; Wiznitzer, A.; Sergienko, R.; Mazor, M.; Holcberg, G.; Sheiner, E. Placental abruption: Critical analysis of risk factors and perinatal outcomes. *J. Matern. Fetal Neonatal Med.* **2011**, *24*, 698–702. [CrossRef]

27. Walfisch, A.; Sheiner, E. Placenta previa and immediate outcome of the term offspring. *Arch. Gynecol. Obstet.* **2016**, *294*, 739–744. [CrossRef]
28. Schwarzman, P.; Sheiner, E.; Wainstock, T.; Mastrolia, S.A.; Segal, I.; Landau, D.; Walfisch, A. Vacuum Extraction in Preterm Deliveries and Long-Term Neurological Outcome of the Offspring. *Pediatr. Neurol.* **2019**, *94*, 55–60. [CrossRef]
29. Parker, S.E.; Werler, M.M. Epidemiology of ischemic placental disease: A focus on preterm gestations. *Semin. Perinatol.* **2014**, *38*, 133–138. [CrossRef]
30. Chisholm, K.M.; Norton, M.E.; Penn, A.A.; Heerema-McKenney, A. Classification of Preterm Birth With Placental Correlates. *Pediatr. Dev. Pathol.* **2018**, *21*, 548–560. [CrossRef]
31. Garmi, G.; Okopnik, M.; Keness, Y.; Zafran, N.; Berkowitz, E.; Salim, R. Correlation between Clinical, Placental Histology and Microbiological Findings in Spontaneous Preterm Births. *Fetal Diagn. Ther.* **2016**, *40*, 141–149. [CrossRef]
32. Tikkanen, M. Placental abruption: Epidemiology, risk factors and consequences. *Acta Obstet. Gynecol. Scand.* **2011**, *90*, 140–149. [CrossRef]
33. Lao, T. Does Maternal Glucose Intolerance Affect the Length of Gestation in Singleton Pregnancies? *J. Soc. Gynecol. Eval.* **2003**, *10*, 366–371. [CrossRef]
34. Sibai, B.M.; Caritis, S.N.; Hauth, J.C.; MacPherson, C.; VanDorsten, J.P.; Klebanoff, M.; Landon, M.; Paul, R.H.; Meis, P.J.; Miodovnik, M.; et al. Preterm delivery in women with pregestational diabetes mellitus or chronic hypertension relative to women with uncomplicated pregnancies. *Am. J. Obstet. Gynecol.* **2000**, *183*, 1520–1524. [CrossRef]
35. Hendler, I.; Goldenberg, R.L.; Mercer, B.M.; Iams, J.D.; Meis, P.J.; Moawad, A.H.; MacPherson, C.A.; Caritis, S.N.; Miodovnik, M.; Menard, K.M.; et al. The Preterm Prediction Study: Association between maternal body mass index and spontaneous and indicated preterm birth. *Am. J. Obstet. Gynecol.* **2005**, *192*, 882–886. [CrossRef]
36. Yang, J.; Baer, R.J.; Berghella, V.; Chambers, C.; Chung, P.; Coker, T.; Currier, R.J.; Druzin, M.L.; Kuppermann, M.; Muglia, L.J.; et al. Recurrence of Preterm Birth and Early Term Birth. *Obstet. Gynecol.* **2016**, *128*, 364–372. [CrossRef]

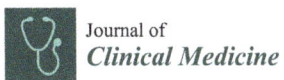

Article

Can We Predict Preterm Delivery Based on the Previous Pregnancy?

Tamar Wainstock [1,*], Ruslan Sergienko [1] and Eyal Sheiner [2]

[1] Department of Public Health, Faculty of Health Sciences, Ben-Gurion University of the Negev, Beer-Sheva 8489325, Israel; sergienk@bgu.ac.il

[2] Department of Obstetrics and Gynecology, Soroka University Medical Center, Ben-Gurion University of the Negev, Beer-Sheva 8489325, Israel; sheiner@bgu.ac.il

* Correspondence: wainstoc@bgu.ac.il; Tel.: +972-523114880

Abstract: (1) Background: Preterm deliveries (PTD, <37 gestational weeks) which occur in 5–18% of deliveries across the world, are associated with immediate and long-term offspring morbidity, as well as high costs to health systems. Our aim was to identify risk factors during the first pregnancy ending at term for PTD in the subsequent pregnancy. (2) Methods: A retrospective population-based nested case–control study was conducted, including all women with two first singleton consecutive deliveries. Women with PTD in the first pregnancy were excluded. Characteristics and complications of the first pregnancy were compared among cases, defined as women with PTD in their second pregnancy, and the controls, defined as women delivering at term in their second pregnancy. A multivariable logistic regression model was used to study the association between pregnancy complications (in the first pregnancy) and PTD (in the subsequent pregnancy), while adjusting for maternal age and the interpregnancy interval. (3) Results: A total of 39,780 women were included in the study, 5.2% (n = 2088) had PTD in their second pregnancy. Women with PTD, as compared to controls (i.e., delivered at term in second pregnancy), were more likely to have the following complications in their first pregnancy: perinatal mortality (0.4% vs. 1.0%), small for gestational age (12.4% vs. 8.1%), and preeclampsia (7.6% vs. 5.7%). In the multivariable model, after adjusting for maternal age, interpregnancy interval and co-morbidities, having any one of these first pregnancy complications was independently associated with an increased risk for PTD (adjusted OR = 1.44; 95%CI 1.28–1.62), and the risk was greater if two or more complications were diagnosed (adjusted OR = 2.09; 95%CI 1.47–3.00). These complications were also risk factors for early PTD (<34 gestational weeks), PTD with a systematic infectious disease in the background, and possibly with spontaneous PTD. (4) Conclusions: First pregnancy complications are associated with an increased risk for PTD in the subsequent pregnancy. First pregnancy, although ending at term, may serve as a window of opportunity to identify women at risk for future PTD.

Keywords: perinatal mortality; preeclampsia; pregnancy complications; preterm birth; preterm delivery; small for gestational age

1. Introduction

Preterm delivery (PTD), defined as delivery before 37 complete gestational weeks [1], is the main cause for newborn death and childhood disability and the second cause of death in children up to the age of five years [2]. PTD rates vary by country, ranging in recent years from ~5% in European countries, 9.6% in the USA and 18% in some African countries [3,4]. In most countries, PTD rates are increasing, and an estimated 15 million babies (11.1% of live births), are born premature worldwide every year [2,3,5].

Fetal development occurs throughout the entire pregnancy until full term, therefore, when PTD occurs, the newborn is not physiologically and metabolically mature, leading to immediate and long term complications [3]. Risk and severity of these complications depend mainly on gestational age at delivery and increase with reduced gestational age.

The causes for PTD are mainly unknown, and they are usually multifactorial, including genetic factors, utero-placental dysfunction or underlying inflammation processes [6].

PTD risk factors, including subtypes of PTD, have been extensively studied. The leading PTD risk factor is having a history of PTD [7–10]. The risk increases with each additional PTD in a woman's history, or if the PTD occurred in the immediately preceding pregnancy, and with earlier gestational age at the previous PTD [7].

It is recommended for women with a history of PTD to receive more intensive prenatal monitoring, including treatment strategies to reduce PTD risk. Often weekly mid-trimester 17-alpha-hydroxyprogesterone caproate (17-OHPC) are applied to reduce risk for PTD recurrence [11,12].

A history of pregnancy complications in term pregnancies has also been suggested to be associated with subsequent pregnancy PTD risk [13–15]. These complications mainly include threatened PTD, small for gestational age (SGA) and perinatal mortality. Less is known, however, regarding the risk factors by the type of PTD and by the extremity of the PTD.

Since a history of PTD is a main risk factor for its recurrence, the aim of the current study was to identify additional PTD risk factors, among a population of women without a history of PTD. Specifically, the risk factors were studied among women with spontaneous PTD, early PTD (<34 gestational weeks), and PTD with an infectious disease in the background (with a possible inflammatory etiology).

2. Experimental Section

The study was conducted at the Soroka University Medical Center (SUMC) located in the Southern region of Israel. SUMC, the single tertiary medical center in the region, serves a population of >1 million residents, and has the country's largest birthing center with approximately 17,000 yearly births in recent years.

The study protocol received the SUMC IRB approval (#0355819SOR, October 2019), and informed consent was exempt.

A retrospective population-based nested case–control study was conducted. Inclusion criteria: All women with two first singleton consecutive deliveries between the years 1988–2017. Exclusion criteria: Women with PTD in the first pregnancy, multiple gestations (in either pregnancy). Cases were defined as women with PTD in their second pregnancy, and they were compared to the controls, defined as women delivering at term in their second pregnancy. Primary outcomes: Characteristics and complications of the first pregnancy, which were compared among cases and controls.

First pregnancy characteristics and complications that were significantly different between cases and controls were included in the multivariable analysis. Multivariable logistic regression models were used to study the association between pregnancy complications (in the first pregnancy) and PTD (in the subsequent pregnancy), while adjusting for maternal age (3 categories: <20; 20–35; ≥35) and interpregnancy interval (3 categories: <6 months; 6 months- 5 years; ≥5 years). The interpregnancy interval was defined as the time between first delivery and best estimation of first day of last menstruation period of the second pregnancy, based on clinical evaluation and first trimester sonar test. Interpregnancy interval, either short or long, has been associated with increased risk for several adverse pregnancy outcomes, including small for gestational age (SGA, defined as birthweight < 5th percentile for gestational age and sex), low birthweight (<2500 g), PTD and perinatal death [16–20]. It has also been shown to affect offspring long-term health [21,22]. The short interpregnancy interval may not allow the mother enough time to recuperate physiologically from the previous pregnancy and birth, and increase the risk for SGA and PTD. A long interpregnancy interval is associated with older maternal age, obesity and increased incidence of secondary infertility, morbidities and pregnancy complications.

A combined adverse pregnancy score was created, which summed the following first pregnancy complications (which were associated with second pregnancy preterm birth, based on the first step analysis): SGA, perinatal mortality or preeclampsia (defined as either of the following ICD-9 codes: 642.41; 642.42; 642.51; 642.52; 642.61; 642.62). Scoring of this variable ranged between 0 = no complications; 1 = one complication, 2 = two or more complications. A multivariable logistic model was then used to study whether the risk for PTD in the second pregnancy increased with each first pregnancy complication, and for each additional complication, based on the combined adverse pregnancy score. Women without first pregnancy complications were defined as the reference group.

In order to evaluate how early the second pregnancy PTD occurred following the first pregnancy complications, the mean (±standard deviation, SD) of gestational ages among the cases were evaluated regarding each first pregnancy complication.

Several subanalyses were performed that were:

1. Aiming to study risk factors for spontaneous PTD, the incidence of first pregnancy complications was compared between term deliveries and cases of spontaneous PTD in the second pregnancy. Spontaneous PTD included the following diagnoses: spontaneous premature rupture of the membranes or premature contractions (ICD-9 codes: 651.1; 644.21, respectively). Excluded were all cases of indicated PTD or PTD of a nondefinite nature (they may have been either spontaneous or indicated), which had the following diagnoses: placental abruption (ICD-9 code: 641.21), fetal growth restriction, preeclampsia (ICD-9 codes: 642.41, 642.51, 642.61, 642.62, 642.42, 642.52), meconium stained amniotic fluid (ICD-9 code 656.81), chronic hypertension (ICD-9 code 642.01), polyhydramnios (ICD-9 code 657.01), oligohydramnios (ICD-9 code 658.01), or pathological presentation (breech, transverse of face, ICD-9 codes 652.81, 652.21, 652.31, 652.41, 660.31).

2. Aiming to study risk factors for early PTD (<34 weeks), a more severe outcome with greater complications to the offspring, incidence of first pregnancy complications was compared between term deliveries and cases of early PTD in second pregnancy. Women who delivered between 34.0–36.99 gestational week were excluded.

3. Aiming to study risk factors for PTD involving an infectious etiology, incidence of first pregnancy complications was compared between term deliveries and PTD cases involving an infection etiology in the second pregnancy. Systematic infection was defined as having either of the following, prior to the PTD: bacterial or viral infections, of known or unknown causes, including pneumonia, urinary tract infections, endometritis, etc.

The multivariable analysis with the combined adverse score was performed for each of the subanalyses.

3. Results

A total of 39,780 women were included in the study, 5.2% (n = 2088) delivered preterm in their second pregnancy (i.e., cases). Of them, the incidence of definite spontaneous PTD (following premature rupture of the membranes or contractions) was 14.8% (n = 310) and incidence of indicated PTB (following premature rupture of the membranes, fetal growth restriction or preeclampsia) was 15.2% (n = 318).

Table 1 presents a comparison of the participants' characteristics, as well as first and second pregnancy characteristics, between cases and controls. As can be seen, cases were slightly older, delivered heavier newborns, and were more likely to have the following complications in their first pregnancy: perinatal mortality (1.0% vs. 0.4%; OR = 2.56 95%CI 1.60–4.09, $p < 0.001$), small for gestational age (SGA, 12.4% vs. 8.1%; OR = 1.60 95%CI 1.39–1.83, $p < 0.001$), preeclampsia (7.6% vs. 5.7%; OR = 1.34 95%CI 1.14–1.59, $p < 0.001$) and offspring with low birthweight (LBW, birthweight <2500 gr.: 12.3% vs. 5.7%; OR = 2.31; 2.01–2.65, $p < 0.001$). Rates of gestational diabetes, placental abruption and cesarean deliveries were comparable between the groups. Among the cases of first pregnancy perinatal mortality, the possible causes of the mortality did not differ between the cases and the controls, for instance: 7 (35%) versus 44 (31%) were diagnosed with chromosomal abnormalities or malformations among cases and controls, respectively, and intrauterine fetal death 11 (55.0%) versus 72 (50.7%) among cases and controls, respectively.

Table 1. Maternal, first and second pregnancy characteristics by cases and controls.

	Cases (PTD Second Pregnancy) n = 2088 (5.2%)	Controls (Term Second Pregnancy) n = 37,692 (94.8%)	p-Value
Maternal Characteristics			
Ethnicity			<0.001
Jewish	928 (4.4)	20,036 (95.6)	
Bedouin	1160 (6.2)	17,656 (93.8)	
Smoking	23 (1.1)	458 (1.2)	0.75
Chronic hypertension	32 (1.5)	217 (0.6)	<0.001
Diabetes mellitus	13 (0.6)	90 (0.2)	0.003
First Pregnancy Characteristics			
Maternal age (mean ± SD)	23.39 ± 4.0	22.72 ± 4.2	<0.001
<20	393 (18.9)	4564 (12.1)	<0.001
20–35	1624 (78.0)	32,231 (85.6)	
≥35	65 (3.1)	843 (2.2)	
Birthweight (mean ± SD)	3139 ± 416	2961 ± 425	<0.001
Gestational age (mean ± SD)	38.93 ± 1.30	39.49 ± 1.25	<0.001
First and second pregnancy interval mean ± SD)	1.56 ± 1.52	1.47 ± 1.75	0.03
<6 months	582 (27.9)	7550 (20.0)	<0.001
between 6 months and 5 years	1414 (67.7)	28,810 (76.4)	
≥5 years	92 (4.4)	1332 (3.5)	
			Odds ratio; 95%CI, p-value
Fertility treatments *	60 (2.9)	1043 (2.8)	1.04; 0.8–1.35, 0.74
Obesity *	10 (0.5)	275 (0.7)	0.66; 0.35–1.23, 0.23
Cesarean delivery	241 (11.5)	4494 (11.9)	0.96; 0.84–1.10, 0.62
full dilatation cesarean sections	44 (18.3)	596 (13.3)	1.46; 1.04–2.05, 0.03
Low Apgar (<7) at 5 min	9 (0.4)	179 (0.5)	0.91; 0.47–1.79, 1.0
Perinatal mortality	20 (1.0)	142 (0.4)	2.56; 1.60–4.09, <0.001
Low birthweight (<2500 gr.)	256 (12.3)	2148 (5.7)	2.31; 2.01–2.65, <0.001
Chromosomal abnormalities or congenital malformations	130 (6.2)	2065 (5.5)	1.14; 0.95–1.37, =0.15
Small for gestational age *	258 (12.4)	3059 (8.1)	1.60; 1.39–1.83, <0.001
Mild or severe preeclampsia or eclampsia	158 (7.6)	2165 (5.7)	1.34; 1.14–1.59, <0.001
Gestational diabetes	67 (3.2)	1096 (2.9)	1.11; 0.86–1.42, 0.43
Placental abruption	9 (0.4)	100 (0.3)	1.63; 0.82–3.22, 0.19
Prolonged first stage of delivery	38 (1.8)	1031 (2.7)	0.66; 0.47–0.91, 0.012
Prolonged second stage of delivery	81 (3.9)	1401 (3.7)	1.04; 0.83–1.31, 0.68
Second Pregnancy Characteristics			
Preeclampsia	110 (5.3)	764 (2.0)	2.69; 2.19–3.30, <0.001
Fetal growth restriction	161 (7.7)	504 (1.3)	6.16; 5.13–7.40, <0.001
Placenta abruption	75 (3.6)	84 (0.2)	16.68; 12.18–22.85, <0.001
Rupture of the membranes	300 (14.4)	2518 (6.7)	2.34; 2.06–2.67, <0.001

* Fertility treatments: including ovulation induction or in vitro fertilization; obesity: BMI > 30; small for gestational age: birthweight < 5th percentile for gestational age and gender.

In the second pregnancy, the incidence of preeclampsia, fetal growth restriction and placental abruption were all higher among the pregnancies ending with PTD as compared to term deliveries.

In three multivariable models (not presented), which adjusted for categories of maternal age in second pregnancy and interpregnancy interval, first pregnancy with either SGA (adjusted OR = 1.54; 95%CI 1.35–1.77, $p < 0.001$), preeclampsia (adjusted OR = 1.36; 95%CI 1.15–1.61, $p = 0.001$) or perinatal mortality (adjusted OR = 2.27; 95%CI 1.41–3.64, $p < 0.001$), was independently associated with second pregnancy PTD risk. A combined adverse first pregnancy outcome variable was created, including the sum of the following diagnoses:

SGA, perinatal mortality and preeclampsia (scoring 0, 1, ≥2). In the multivariable model presented in Table 2, having a history of any one of the complications was independently associated with an increased risk for PTD (adjusted OR = 1.46; 95%CI 1.30–1.65, $p < 0.001$), and the risk was greater if two or more complications were diagnosed (adjusted OR = 2.20; 95%CI 1.54–3.13, $p < 0.001$). The model was adjusted for maternal age, interpregnancy interval, maternal comorbidities and year of delivery.

Table 2. Multivariable analysis for the association between first pregnancy complications and PTD risk in second pregnancy.

Variable	Adjusted Odds Ratio; 95%CI	p
Any adverse first pregnancy outcome (vs. none) *	1.44; 1.28–1.62	<0.001
Any two or three complications (vs. none)	2.09; 1.47–3.00	<0.001
Maternal age		
<20	1.56; 1.38–1.75	<0.001
20–35	1 (Ref.)	
≥35	1.16; 0.91–1.48	0.216
Interpregnancy interval		
<6 months	1.44; 1.30–1.60	<0.001
between 6 months and 5 years	1 (Ref.)	
≥5 years	1.44; 1.15–1.80	0.001
delivery year	1.0; 0.99–1.00	0.459
obesity	0.81; 0.29–2.27	0.694
chronic high blood pressure	2.53; 1.73–3.70	<0.001
diabetes	2.65; 1.46–4.79	0.001

* The following complications were included: SGA, perinatal mortality or preeclampsia.

The distribution of gestational ages among PTD in second pregnancy, by first pregnancy complication were as follow: among pregnancies with SGA 33.81 ± 3.1; among pregnancies with preeclampsia 34.2 ± 3.1; and among PTD following pregnancies with perinatal mortality 33.2 ± 3.7.

There were 310 (14.8%) definite spontaneous PTD and 318 (15.2%) cases of indicated PTD. In the subanalysis, cases of spontaneous PTD were compared to the control group (term delivery). The incidence of first pregnancy SGA, perinatal mortality and preeclampsia were all higher among the spontaneous PTD group, the differences were not statistically significant, most likely due to the small sample size (SGA: 11.9% versus 9.0%, OR = 1.36, 95%CI 0.98–1.99, $p = 0.071$, perinatal mortality: 0.6% versus 0.4%, OR = 1.72; 95%CI 0.42–6.96, $p = 0.33$, preeclampsia: 6.1% versus 5.7%, OR = 1.07; 95%CI 0.67–1.71, $p = 0.73$). A combined adverse first pregnancy outcome variable was created, including any of the following diagnoses: SGA, perinatal mortality or preeclampsia (scoring 0 or 1). The incidence of having at least one complication in the first pregnancy was 19.0% versus 15.4% among the spontaneous PTD versus the term pregnancies, respectively, (OR = 1.29, 95%CI 0.97–1.72, $p = 0.08$). In the multivariable analysis (presented in Table 3), while adjusting for maternal age and interpregnancy intervals, first term delivery with either SGA, perinatal mortality or preeclampsia, was associated with an increased risk for spontaneous subsequent pregnancy PTD (adjusted OR = 1.29, 95%CI 0.97–1.72, $p = 0.078$). This finding was not statistically significant, however the possibility that the findings were due to insufficient power cannot be ruled out (Power = 39%).

There were 543 (1.4%) cases of early preterm (gestational age < 34) in second delivery, compared to term deliveries. First pregnancy incidence of SGA (13.6% versus 8.3%, OR = 1.75, 95%CI 1.37–2.24, $p < 0.001$) and perinatal mortality (1.1% versus 0.4%, OR = 2.80, 95%CI 1.23–6.35, $p = 0.024$) were both significantly higher among women with second pregnancy early preterm delivery. The incidence of preeclampsia was slightly higher (6.6% versus 5.8%, OR = 1.5, 95%CI 0.82–1.61) among this group. Among mothers without a history of any complications, the risk for early PTD was 1.3%, and the risk was 2.3% and 3.2% among mothers with one and two complications, respectively (p for trend < 0.001). In the multivariable analysis (presented in Table 3), while adjusting for maternal age and interpregnancy intervals, first term delivery with either SGA, perinatal mortality or preeclampsia, was associated with an increased risk for early subsequent pregnancy PTD (adjusted OR = 1.73; 1.42–2.11, $p < 0.001$).

Table 3. Multivariable analysis for the association between first pregnancy complications and PTD risk in second pregnancy.

Variable	Spontaneous PTD Only		Early PTD Only		PTD Following a Systemic Infectious Disease	
	Adjusted Odds Ratio; 95%CI	p	Adjusted Odds Ratio; 95%CI	p	Adjusted Odds Ratio; 95%CI	p
Any adverse first pregnancy outcome (vs. none) *	1.29; 0.97–1.72	0.078	1.73; 1.42–2.11	<0.001	1.63; 1.17–2.28	0.004
Maternal age						
<20	0.99; 0.7–1.42	0.98	2.06; 1.67–2.54	<0.001	1.51; 1.05–2.17	0.027
20–35	1 (Ref.)		1 (Ref.)		1 (Ref.)	
≥35	1.41; 0.83–2.38	0.20	1.51; 0.99–2.32	0.06	0.97; 0.45–2.11	0.95
Interpregnancy interval (years)						
<6 months	0.95; 0.71–1.28	0.75	1.39; 1.15–1.70	0.002	1.13; 0.82–1.57	0.45
between 6 months and 5 years	1 (Ref.)		1 (Ref.)		1 (Ref.)	
≥5 years	1.64; 1.01–2.66	0.047	1.36; 0.88–2.12	0.16	1.46; 0.76–2.83	0.26

* The following complications were included: SGA, perinatal mortality or preeclampsia.

There were 215 (8.8% of all PTDs) PTD second deliveries with systematic infectious disease in the background, compared to 37,692 term deliveries. Among this group 40 (18.6%) had definite spontaneous delivery. First pregnancy incidence of SGA (11.6% versus 8.1%, OR = 1.49, 95%CI 0.98–2.26, $p = 0.073$), perinatal mortality (1.9% versus 0.4%, OR = 5.01, 95%CI 1.84–13.67, $p = 0.01$) and preeclampsia (9.8% versus 5.7%, OR = 1.78, 95%CI 1.13–2.79, $p = 0.018$) were all higher among the cases with second pregnancy PTD with systematic infectious disease in the background. Among mothers without a history of any complications, the risk for PTD with systematic infectious disease in the background was 0.5%, and the risk was 0.8% and 2.0%, among mothers with any one or ≥2 complications, respectively (p for trend < 0.001). In the multivariable analysis (presented in Table 3), while adjusting for maternal age and interpregnancy intervals, first term delivery with either SGA, perinatal mortality or preeclampsia, was associated with an increased risk for PTD in second pregnancy with systematic infectious disease in the background (adjusted OR= 1.63; 1.17–2.28, $p = 0.004$).

4. Discussion

In this large population-based retrospective nested case−control study, first term pregnancy complicated with either SGA, preeclampsia or perinatal mortality, was associated with an increased risk for PTD in the subsequent pregnancy. These findings were also true specifically for early PTD, PTD with a possible inflammatory etiology, or spontaneous PTD, although the later was without statistical significance. This association was independent of maternal age, interpregnancy interval and maternal comorbidities. Exposure to more than one of these first pregnancy complications was associated with an even greater risk.

First pregnancy complications were associated with not only late, near term PTD, but also with extreme PTD: while the majority of second pregnancy PTD occurred between gestational ages 35–36, among women with a first pregnancy which ended with perinatal mortality, 25% of PTD deliveries occurred at <32 gestational weeks; and in nearly 40% of women with first pregnancy SGA, the PTD occurred at <34 gestational weeks. The associations between the first pregnancy complications were weaker regarding spontaneous PTD, which suggest other risk factors are relevant in these cases, however the possibility of lack of power to detect such differences cannot be ruled out.

Findings of the current study are in agreement with previous studies that found that women with a history of term SGA or fetal mortality were at increased risk for PTD [13]. The strongest risk factor of PTD is a previous PTD, therefore chronic environmental [23–25], and genetic factors are most likely involved in PTD etiology [26,27]. The current study addresses first PTD occurrence and its association with previous term pregnancy SGA, preeclampsia and perinatal mortality, all of which may be due to several mechanisms and causes. These four complications may share similar mechanisms, and therefore reoccur in the same mother, and can serve as markers of increased risk for the other complications [28].

The underlining cause and mechanism of PTD is not yet completely understood, and even less is known regarding causes of spontaneous PTD. The main mechanisms that have been suggested are inflammation, infection, and vascular pathologies [29,30]. Usually multiple etiologies are involved, including: cervical insufficiency, decline in progesterone action and insufficiency or ischemic placental–uterine unit [29,31,32]. Impaired placental implantation processes and insufficient fetal nutrition and growth may cause deliveries of SGA newborns, preeclampsia, perinatal mortality, placental abruption and PTD [33,34]. In the current study, placental abruption in the second pregnancy was a risk factor for PTD in the second pregnancy, but having a history of term placental abruption was not a risk factor.

An inflammatory process has been suggested as a main factor in PTD, causing premature contractions and (mainly) spontaneous PTD [35]. In our study, women delivering preterm with an infectious disease in the background, have also presented with higher rates of SGA, preeclampsia and perinatal mortality in the first pregnancy. Although it is not clear whether neonatal outcomes are affected by the maternal infection [36], it is possible women with an infectious disease during pregnancy, and with a history of these complications, would benefit from PTD prevention strategies.

Several study limitations need to be addressed. Since this was a retrospective cohort and based on medical records, data regarding additional potential confounding variables was unavailable, such as environmental and life-style characteristics, and may have caused a residual confounding effect. However, since this was a large population-based study, in which the two pregnancies of each mother were matched and compared, it can be expected that familial, background and environmental factors were relatively similar between the two pregnancies, and in case of a distortion of the true association existed, it was minimal.

The aim in the current study was to identify second pregnancy PTD risk factors during the first pregnancy, and therefore the current findings are not valid or relevant for PTD risk among primiparous women or for PTD recurrence. Still, according to our findings, initial PTD occurred in 5.2% of second pregnancies, therefore this is a relatively prevalent pregnancy complication, to which our findings are relevant.

It is possible women with previous pregnancy complications were under more frequent and closer monitoring and were therefore more likely to be diagnosed with second pregnancy complications, leading to a higher incidence of indicated PTD among this group. However, a subanalysis among spontaneous second pregnancy PTD showed similar results, suggesting detection bias is unlikely.

PTD is a major cause of death and a significant cause of long-term morbidities and disabilities, and the risks are greater with decreasing gestational age at delivery. Lowering the rate of this major pregnancy complication has been declared by the World Health Organization as "an urgent priority for reaching the Millennium Development Goal, calling for the reduction of child deaths" [2]. While risk factors for PTD have been widely studied, and although strategies and diagnostic tools to prevent PTD have been practised for over 30 years, the expectations have not been met and PTD rates have not declined. Some PTD risk factors are preventable, and addressing them, in the personal and population levels, may decrease PTD risk. Even a small reduction in PTD can have a large public health and economic impact, both in terms of preventing perinatal mortality, morbidity and lifelong disability among affected infants.

5. Conclusions

First pregnancy complications are associated with an increased risk for PTD in the subsequent pregnancy, and specifically with PTD with maternal infectious disease in the background, early PTDs, and possible spontaneous PTDs. First pregnancy, although ending at term, may serve as a window of opportunity to identify women at risk for future PTD, and PTD prevention strategies which are recommended for women with a history of PTD, should be considered for women with history of these other pregnancy complications.

Author Contributions: Conceptualization, T.W. and E.S.; methodology, T.W. and E.S.; software, R. S. and T.W.; formal analysis, T.W. and R.S.; writing—original draft preparation, T.W.; writing—review and editing, E.S. All authors have read and agreed to the published version of the manuscript.

Funding: This research received no external funding.

Institutional Review Board Statement: The study was conducted according to the guidelines of the Declaration of Helsinki, and approved by the Institutional Review Board of Soroka University Medical Center (protocol #0355819SOR, October 2019).

Informed Consent Statement: Patient consent was waived due to the de-identified computerized data-based nature of the study.

Data Availability Statement: Data will be available by request and according to the IRB restrictions.

Conflicts of Interest: The authors declare no conflict of interest.

References

1. CDC. Available online: https//www.cdc.gov/reproductivehealth/MaternalInfantHealth/PretermBirth.html (accessed on 30 March 2021).
2. WHO. Available online: https://www.who.int/news-room/fact-sheets/detail/preterm-birth (accessed on 30 March 2021).
3. Blencowe, H.; Cousens, S.; Oestergaard, M.Z.; Chou, D.; Moller, A.B.; Narwal, R.; Lawn, J.E. National, regional and worldwide estimates of preterm birth. *Lancet* **2012**, *379*, 2162–2172. [CrossRef]
4. Hamilton, B.E.; Martin, J.A.; Osterman, M.J.; Curtin, S.C.; Matthews, T.J. Births, Final Data for 2014. *Natl. Vital Stat. Rep.* **2015**, *64*, 1–64. [PubMed]
5. Blencowe, H.; Cousens, S.; Chou, D.; Oestergaard, M.; Say, L.; Moller, A.-B.; Kinney, M.; Lawn, J.; the Born Too Soon Preterm Birth Action Group (see acknowledgement for full list). Born Too Soon: The global epidemiology of 15 million preterm births. *Reprod. Heal.* **2013**, *10*, S2. [CrossRef]
6. Romero, R.; Dey, S.K.; Fisher, S.J. Preterm labor, one syndrome, many causes. *Science* **2014**, *345*, 760–765. [CrossRef]
7. Mercer, B.M.; Goldenberg, R.L.; Moawad, A.H.; Meis, P.J.; Iams, J.D.; Das, A.F.; National Institute of Child Health Human Development Maternal-Fetal Medicine Units Network The preterm prediction study, effect of gestational age and cause of preterm birth on subsequent obstetric outcome. National Institute of Child Health and Human Development Maternal-Fetal Medicine Units Network. *Am. J. Obstet. Gynecol.* **1999**, *181 Pt 1*, 1216–1221. [CrossRef]
8. Yang, J.; Baer, R.J.; Berghella, V.; Chambers, C.; Chung, P.; Coker, T.; Currier, R.J.; Druzin, M.L.; Kuppermann, M.; Muglia, L.J.; et al. Recurrence of Preterm Birth and Early Term Birth. *Obstet. Gynecol.* **2016**, *128*, 364–372. [CrossRef]
9. Laughon, S.K.; Albert, P.S.; Leishear, K.; Mendola, P. The NICHD Consecutive Pregnancies Study: Recurrent preterm delivery by subtype. *Am. J. Obstet. Gynecol.* **2014**, *210*, 131.e1–131.e8. [CrossRef]
10. Mazaki-Tovi, S.; Romero, R.; Kusanovic, J.P.; Erez, O.; Pineles, B.L.; Gotsch, F.; Mittal, P.; Than, N.G.; Espinoza, J.; Hassan, S.S. Recurrent Preterm Birth. *Semin. Perinatol.* **2007**, *31*, 142–158. [CrossRef] [PubMed]
11. Meis, P.J.; Klebanoff, M.; Thom, E.; Dombrowski, M.P.; Sibai, B.; Moawad, A.H.; Spong, C.Y.; Hauth, J.C.; Miodovnik, M.; Varner, M.W.; et al. Prevention of Recurrent Preterm Delivery by 17 Alpha-Hydroxyprogesterone Caproate. *N. Engl. J. Med.* **2003**, *348*, 2379–2385. [CrossRef] [PubMed]
12. Fernandez-Macias, R.; Martinez-Portilla, R.J.; Cerrillos, L.; Figueras, F.; Palacio, M. A systematic review and meta-analysis of randomized controlled trials comparing 17-alpha-hydroxyprogesterone caproate versus placebo for the prevention of recurrent preterm birth. *Int. J. Gynecol. Obstet.* **2019**, *147*, 156–164. [CrossRef]
13. Baer, R.J.; Berghella, V.; Muglia, L.J.; Norton, M.E.; Rand, L.; Ryckman, K.K.; Jelliffe-Pawlowski, L.L.; McLemore, M.R. Previous Adverse Outcome of Term Pregnancy and Risk of Preterm Birth in Subsequent Pregnancy. *Matern. Child Heal. J.* **2018**, *23*, 443–450. [CrossRef]
14. Wong, L.F.; Wilkes, J.; Korgenski, K.; Varner, M.W.; Manuck, T.A. Risk factors associated with preterm birth after a prior term delivery. *BJOG: Int. J. Obstet. Gynaecol.* **2016**, *123*, 1772–1778. [CrossRef]
15. Cho, G.J.; Choi, S.-J.; Lee, K.-M.; Han, S.W.; Kim, H.Y.; Ahn, K.-H.; Hong, S.-C.; Kim, H.-J.; Oh, M.-J. Women with threatened preterm labour followed by term delivery have an increased risk of spontaneous preterm birth in subsequent pregnancies: A population-based cohort study. *BJOG Int. J. Obstet. Gynaecol.* **2019**, *126*, 901–905. [CrossRef]
16. Conde-Agudelo, A.; Rosas-Bermúdez, A.; Kafury-Goeta, A.C. Birth Spacing and Risk of Adverse Perinatal Outcomes. *JAMA* **2006**, *295*, 1809–1823. [CrossRef]

17. Grisaru-Granovsky, S.; Gordon, E.-S.; Haklai, Z.; Samueloff, A.; Schimmel, M.M. Effect of interpregnancy interval on adverse perinatal outcomes—A national study. *Contracept.* **2009**, *80*, 512–518. [CrossRef]
18. DeFranco, E.A.; Stamilio, D.M.; Boslaugh, S.E.; Gross, G.A.; Muglia, L.J. A short interpregnancy interval is a risk factor for preterm birth and its recurrence. *Am. J. Obstet. Gynecol.* **2007**, *197*, 264.e1–264.e6. [CrossRef] [PubMed]
19. Zhu, B.-P.; Rolfs, R.T.; Nangle, B.E.; Horan, J.M. Effect of the Interval between Pregnancies on Perinatal Outcomes. *N. Engl. J. Med.* **1999**, *340*, 589–594. [CrossRef] [PubMed]
20. DeFranco, E.A.; Seske, L.M.; Greenberg, J.M.; Muglia, L.J. Influence of interpregnancy interval on neonatal morbidity. *Am. J. Obstet. Gynecol.* **2015**, *212*, 386.e1–386.e9. [CrossRef]
21. Elhakham, D.; Wainstock, T.; Sheiner, E.; Sergienko, R.; Pariente, G. Inter-pregnancy interval and long-term neurological morbidity of the offspring. *Arch. Gynecol. Obstet.* **2021**, *303*, 703–708. [CrossRef] [PubMed]
22. Imterat, M.; Wainstock, T.; Sheiner, E.; Pariente, G. Inter-pregnancy interval and later pediatric cardiovascular health of the offspring—A population-based cohort study. *J. Dev. Orig. Heal. Dis.* **2020**, *2*, 1–5. [CrossRef]
23. Basso, O.; Olsen, J.; Christensen, K. Study of environmental, social, and paternal factors in preterm delivery using sibs and half sibs. A population-based study in Denmark. *J. Epidemiol. Community Health* **1999**, *53*, 20–23. [CrossRef]
24. Li, Q.; Wang, Y.-Y.; Guo, Y.; Zhou, H.; Wang, X.; Wang, Q.; Shen, H.; Zhang, Y.; Yan, D.; Zhang, Y.; et al. Effect of airborne particulate matter of 2.5 μm or less on preterm birth: A national birth cohort study in China. *Environ. Int.* **2018**, *121*, 1128–1136. [CrossRef]
25. Basu, R.; Pearson, D.; Ebisu, K.; Malig, B. Association between PM2.5and PM2.5Constituents and Preterm Delivery in California, 2000–2006. *Paediatr. Périnat. Epidemiol.* **2017**, *31*, 424–434. [CrossRef]
26. Strauss, J.F., 3rd; Romero, R.; Gomez-Lopez, N.; Haymond-Thornburg, H.; Modi, B.P.; Teves, M.E.; Schenkein, H.A. Spontaneous preterm birth, advances toward the discovery of genetic predisposition. *Am. J. Obstet. Gynecol.* **2018**, *218*, 294–314.e2. [CrossRef] [PubMed]
27. Zhang, G.; Feenstra, B.; Bacelis, J.; Julius, J.; Muglia, L.M.; Juodakis, J.; Miller, D.E.; Litterman, N.; Jiang, P.-P.; Russell, L.; et al. Genetic Associations with Gestational Duration and Spontaneous Preterm Birth. *N. Engl. J. Med.* **2017**, *377*, 1156–1167. [CrossRef]
28. Sheiner, E.; Kapur, A.; Retnakaran, R.; Hadar, E.; Poon, L.C.; McIntyre, H.D.; Gooden, R. FIGO (International Federation of Gynecology and Obstetrics) Postpregnancy Initative, Long-term Maternal Implications of Pregnancy Complications—Follow-up Considerations. *Int. J. Gynecol. Obst.* **2019**, *147* (Suppl. 1), 1–31. [CrossRef] [PubMed]
29. Romero, R.; Espinoza, J.; Kusanovic, J.P.; Gotsch, F.; Hassan, S.; Erez, O.; Mazor, M. The preterm parturition syndrome. *BJOG* **2006**, *113* (Suppl. 3), 17–42. [CrossRef]
30. Kessous, R.; Shoham-Vardi, I.; Pariente, G.; Holcberg, G.; Sheiner, E. An association between preterm delivery and long-term maternal cardiovascular morbidity. *Am. J. Obstet. Gynecol.* **2013**, *209*, 368.e1–368.e8. [CrossRef] [PubMed]
31. Clark, E.A.S.; Esplin, S.; Torres, L.; Turok, D.; Yoder, B.A.; Varner, M.W.; Winter, S. Prevention of Recurrent Preterm Birth: Role of the Neonatal Follow-up Program. *Matern. Child Health J.* **2014**, *18*, 858–863. [CrossRef] [PubMed]
32. Tarca, A.L.; Fitzgerald, W.; Chaemsaithong, P.; Xu, Z.; Hassan, S.S.; Grivel, J.; Gomez-Lopez, N.; Panaitescu, B.; Pacora, P.; Maymon, E.; et al. The cytokine network in women with an asymptomatic short cervix and the risk of preterm delivery. *Am. J. Reprod. Immunol.* **2017**, *78*, e12686. [CrossRef] [PubMed]
33. Parker, S.E.; Werler, M.M. Epidemiology of ischemic placental disease: A focus on preterm gestations. *Semin. Perinatol.* **2014**, *38*, 133–138. [CrossRef]
34. Ananth, C.V.; Peltier, M.R.; Chavez, M.R.; Kirby, R.S.; Getahun, D.; Vintzileos, A.M. Recurrence of Ischemic Placental Disease. *Obstet. Gynecol.* **2007**, *110*, 128–133. [CrossRef] [PubMed]
35. Romero, R.; Espinoza, J.; Gonçalves, L.F.; Kusanovic, J.P.; Friel, L.; Hassan, S. The Role of Inflammation and Infection in Preterm Birth. *Semin. Reprod. Med.* **2007**, *25*, 021–039. [CrossRef] [PubMed]
36. Tedesco, R.P.; Galvão, R.B.; Guida, J.P.; Passini-Júnior, R.; Lajos, G.J.; Nomura, M.L.; Rehder, P.M.; Dias, T.Z.; Souza, R.T.; Cecatti, J.G. The role of maternal infection in preterm birth: Evidence from the Brazilian Multicentre Study on Preterm Birth (EMIP). *Clinics* **2020**, *75*, e1508. [CrossRef] [PubMed]

Article

Identification of Vaginal Microbial Communities Associated with Extreme Cervical Shortening in Pregnant Women

Monica Di Paola [1,†], Viola Seravalli [2,†], Sara Paccosi [2], Carlotta Linari [2], Astrid Parenti [2], Carlotta De Filippo [3], Michele Tanturli [4], Francesco Vitali [3], Maria Gabriella Torcia [4,*] and Mariarosaria Di Tommaso [2]

1. Department of Biology, University of Florence, Sesto Fiorentino, 50019 Florence, Italy; monica.dipaola@unifi.it
2. Department of Health Sciences, Division of Obstetrics & Gynecology, University of Florence, 50139 Florence, Italy; viola.seravalli@unifi.it (V.S.); carlotta.linari@unifi.it (C.L.); mariarosaria.ditommaso@unifi.it (M.D.T.); sara.paccosi@unifi.it (S.P.); astrid.parenti@unifi.it (A.P.)
3. Institute of Agricultural Biology and Biotechnology, National Research Council, 56124 Pisa, Italy; carlotta.defilippo@ibba.cnr.it (C.D.F.); francesco.vitali@ibba.cnr.it (F.V.)
4. Department of Experimental and Clinical Medicine, University of Florence, 50139 Florence, Italy; michele.tanturli@unifi.it
* Correspondence: maria.torcia@unifi.it
† These authors contributed equally to this work.

Received: 24 September 2020; Accepted: 6 November 2020; Published: 10 November 2020

Abstract: The vaginal microbiota plays a critical role in pregnancy. Bacteria from *Lactobacillus* spp. are thought to maintain immune homeostasis and modulate the inflammatory responses against pathogens implicated in cervical shortening, one of the risk factors for spontaneous preterm birth. We studied vaginal microbiota in 46 pregnant women of predominantly Caucasian ethnicity diagnosed with short cervix (<25 mm), and identified microbial communities associated with extreme cervical shortening (≤10 mm). Vaginal microbiota was defined by 16S rRNA gene sequencing and clustered into community state types (CSTs), based on dominance or depletion of *Lactobacillus* spp. No correlation between CSTs distribution and maternal age or gestational age was revealed. CST-IV, dominated by aerobic and anaerobic bacteria different than *Lactobacilli*, was associated with extreme cervical shortening (odds ratio (OR) = 15.0, 95% confidence interval (CI) = 1.56–14.21; $p = 0.019$). CST-III (*L. iners*-dominated) was also associated with extreme cervical shortening (OR = 6.4, 95% CI = 1.32–31.03; $p = 0.02$). Gestational diabetes mellitus (GDM) was diagnosed in 10/46 women. Bacterial richness was significantly higher in women experiencing this metabolic disorder, but no association with cervical shortening was revealed by statistical analysis. Our study confirms that *Lactobacillus*-depleted microbiota is significantly associated with an extremely short cervix in women of predominantly Caucasian ethnicity, and also suggests an association between *L. iners*-dominated microbiota (CST III) and cervical shortening.

Keywords: high-risk pregnancy; shortened cervix; microbiome; *Lactobacillus*

1. Introduction

The uterine cervix acts as a physical and immune barrier against pathogens' passage into the uterine cavity during pregnancy. Premature cervical remodeling, shortening, and dilation of the cervix are known risk factors for spontaneous preterm birth (sPTB) [1–4] with the notion that the shorter the cervix, the higher the risk of sPTB [1]. In addition to congenital disorders [5], genetic syndromes (e.g., Ehlers–Danlos syndrome) [6] and progesterone deficiency [7], local inflammation secondary to changes in the cervico-vaginal microbiome is another mechanism that has been proposed to cause cervical shortening [8].

Vaginal microbial communities are largely involved in preventing ascending infections from the vagina into the uterine cavity by pathogens that can seriously compromise pregnancy [9,10]. At least five microbial communities, referred to as community state types (CSTs), have been identified in the vaginal microbiota of healthy reproductive-age non-pregnant women. Four CSTs are dominated by *Lactobacillus* species, better adapted to the vaginal environment [11]. In particular, CST-I is dominated by *Lactobacillus crispatus*, CST-II by *L. gasseri*, CST-III by *L. iners*, CST-V by *L. jensenii*. Each species contributes to the first-line defense against bacterial, fungal, and viral pathogens through the release of antimicrobial and anti-inflammatory products and the production of lactic acid that maintains a low vaginal pH [10,12].

CST-IV is represented by polymicrobial communities that include species belonging to *Gardnerella, Atopobium, Mobiluncus, Megasphoera Prevotella, Streptococcus, Mycoplasma, Ureaplasma, Dialister,* and *Bacteroides* genera [11,13]. CST-IV is more common in African, African-American, and Hispanic women, being detected in 40% to 60% of non-pregnant black women, depending on the country analyzed [10,12,14]. In contrast, the prevalence of CST-IV in Caucasian women is around 10%, as reported in cohorts of non-pregnant women [12,14,15]. High stability of the *Lactobacillus* community was recorded during pregnancy [16,17]. Some reports indicated that the vaginal microbiota is more stable during pregnancy than in non-pregnant women [17].

Recent results showed that the vaginal microbiota depleted by *Lactobacillus* spp. (CST-IV) is associated with increased odds of having a short cervix and, that the concomitance of both CST-IV and a short cervix increases the risk of sPTB [8,18]. These results were obtained in a large cohort of pregnant women, mainly of Hispanic, African, African-American ethnicity, whose vaginal microbiota in non-pregnant status is most frequently of the CST-IV type with few to no *Lactobacillus* spp. detected [11,14].

Moreover, metabolic disorders during pregnancy, such as gestational diabetes mellitus (GDM), are known to affect the composition of the vaginal microbiota and the immune homeostasis of the vaginal environment, by being associated with an abundance of potential pathogens and an increase of inflammatory cytokines [19].

In this study, we recruited a cohort of pregnant women (of whom 95% were of Caucasian ethnicity) with sonographic evidence of cervical shortening (<25 mm) revealed in the second or early third trimester of pregnancy. In particular, we aimed to characterize microbial communities associated with cervical length ≤10 mm, which we defined as "extreme cervical shortening", as it has been associated with higher rates of PTB compared to a longer measurement of the cervix (e.g., 20 or 25 mm), at different gestational ages [1,20]. The influence of GDM on vaginal microbiome composition and cervical shortening was also studied.

2. Experimental Section

2.1. Study Population and Sample Collection

The study population consisted of asymptomatic pregnant women with singleton gestation who were referred to the Preterm Birth Clinic of the Department of Obstetrics and Gynecology of Careggi University Hospital (Florence, Italy) between 2014 and 2018 for a cervical length <25 mm in the second or early third trimester (23–32 weeks' gestation). The study was approved by the Ethical Committee of Azienda Ospedaliero-Universitaria Careggi, Firenze (Ref. no. BIO14.0009- 09/07/2014), and all women provided written informed consent. The patients were referred by their obstetricians who detected cervical shortening on a transvaginal ultrasound performed during a routine prenatal visit. Although not under a specific protocol, in private practice in Italy pregnant women are often offered cervical length measurement and this can lead to a diagnosis of a short cervix even after 24–25 weeks of gestation. In some cases, particularly for women who had a cervical length <10 mm, it was the detection of a shortened cervix on a vaginal exam that justified the ultrasound measurement of the cervix.

Exclusion criteria were a history of sPTB, previous surgery to the cervix (cone biopsy and large loop excision), evidence of premature rupture of membranes or symptomatic uterine contractions at the time of recruitment, the presence of fetal abnormalities, vaginal symptoms consistent with infection at the time of enrolment, and the presence of a cervical cerclage or pessary in place at the time of enrolment. All women who are referred to our preterm birth clinic undergo a full obstetric exam and transvaginal ultrasound for assessment of cervical length and a complete medical history is collected by the attending physician. For the purpose of this study, only patients with a singleton gestation and short cervix who did not present any of the exclusion criteria were offered to participate in the study.

Gestational age (GA) was calculated based on the last menstrual period and confirmed by ultrasound. Clinical and demographic information and obstetric history were collected from patients' charts. Repeat measurement of the cervical length by transvaginal ultrasound was performed by trained personnel to confirm cervical shortening at the time of study recruitment. All patients underwent a complete clinical and vaginal examination. Vaginal secretions were collected by inserting a swab approximately 4 to 5 cm into the vagina and gently rotating it several times. The swab was then placed in phosphate-buffered saline (PBS) on ice for 30 min. After swab removal, samples were centrifuged at 8000× g for 10 min, and pellet and supernatant were separately collected and stored at −80 °C. Vaginal progesterone, at a dose of 200 mg daily, was prescribed to 33 patients after sample collection and continued until 34 weeks or until delivery. Placement of a cerclage to prevent PTB in our cohort of patients was not indicated, as "ultrasound-indicated" cerclage in women with short cervix is only considered effective in patients with a history of prior sPTB, which none of our patients had. In addition, none of the patients enrolled in the study received a pessary for prevention of preterm birth after enrollment, either because they did not meet the criteria for pessary placement (cervical length <20 mm before 24 weeks based on our hospital protocol), or because they refused it. On the other hand, women who already had a pessary in place and were referred to the preterm birth clinic for follow-up after discharge from the hospital were considered ineligible for the study, as the impact that the pessary might have on the vaginal microbiota is unknown. All patients were followed until delivery in our preterm birth clinic. Pregnancy and delivery outcomes were collected from patients' charts.

2.2. Bacterial DNA Extraction, 16S Ribosomal RNA Gene Amplicon Preparation, and Illumina MiSeq Sequencing

Bacterial genomic DNA was extracted from the thawed vaginal samples by using the QIAamp DNA Mini Kit (Qiagen, Milano, Italy), following the manufacturer's protocol. Quality control was carried out by gel electrophoresis and measuring ng/µL of DNA by using Qubit 4 Fluorometer (Thermo Fisher Scientific, Milan, Italy) and the related Qubit dsDNA HS (High Sensitivity) assay kit highly selective for double-stranded DNA(Thermo Fisher Scientific, Italy). The library of 16S rRNA gene amplicons was prepared by IGA Technology Services (Udine, Italy) through amplification of the V3-V4 hypervariable region by using specific-barcoded primers with overhanging adapters. The standard protocol was followed according to the 16metagenomic sequencing library preparation guide from Illumina (Part # 15044223 Rev. B; https://support.illumina.com/). Pooled V3-V4 amplicon libraries were sequenced using the Illumina MiSeq platform.

2.3. Sequencing Analysis

The 300-bp paired-end reads obtained from Illumina MiSeq platform for each sample were demultiplexed and quality checked using FastQC 0.11.5. Reads were further processed using the MICCA pipeline (version 1.7.2, http://compmetagen.github.io/micca/) [21] for merging and filtering of reads, chimera checking, and picking of operational taxonomic unit (OTU)/sequence variant (SV), as reported by Meriggi et al. [22]. We obtained 5,705,871 total read counts, with an average per sample equal to 124,040 ± 47,905 (mean ± standard deviation (SD)). Sequence data are available at http://www.ebi.ac.uk/ena/data/view/PRJEB37121, under the accession number PRJEB37121.

2.4. Microbiota Data Analysis

Sequence data analyses were performed in R (v.3.42; R Core Team, 2018), by using phyloseq package v.1.22.3 [23]. Alpha diversity analysis and principal coordinate analysis (PCoA) ordination (beta diversity) based on the Bray–Curtis distances and plots for microbial profile comparison among samples were performed by using the Microbiome Analyst tool (https://www.microbiomeanalyst.ca/) [24], providing OTUs and taxonomy tables and the metadata file. Data filtering was set to remove low-quality features. Considering a total of 1182 OTUs number and 1082 OTUs with ≥2 counts, we fixed the low count filter: minimum count ($n = 2$) and 20% prevalence in samples. Low variance filter: 10% of features removed based on standard deviation. Count data were scaled based on cumulative sum scaling (CSS).

Lactobacillus spp. were assigned based on the Basic Local Alignment Search Tool nucleotide (BLASTn) software (National Center for Biotechnology Information-NCBI database). The highest percentage of identity (Query cover 100% or 99% and Identity 99 or 95%) and expectation value (E-value) was considered to select significant BLAST hits, keeping only outcomes with the lowest E-value (minimal E-value of 10^{-3}). Based on the *Lactobacillus* spp. assignment, Community State Types (CSTs) were defined considering the relative abundance of *Lactobacillus* spp. (>60% in each sample), and aerobic and anaerobic bacteria (ranging from 14 to 40%), as previously indicated [13].

Permutational multivariate analysis of variance (PERMANOVA) and diversity indices calculation (OTU, Shannon, Chao), were calculated using the Microbiome Analyst tool (https://www.microbiomeanalyst.ca/) [24].

To discover potential microbial biomarkers with statistical significance the linear discriminant analysis (LDA) effect size (LEfSe) method was assessed. An alpha significance level of 0.05, either for the factorial Kruskal–Wallis test among classes or for the pairwise Wilcoxon test between subclasses, was used. A size-effect threshold of 2.0 on the logarithmic LDA score was applied for discriminative microbial biomarkers.

2.5. Matrix Metalloproteinase-8 Concentration Measurement

From vaginal fluids, protein concentration was assessed by BCA assay (Euroclone, Milan, Italy). A total of 60 micrograms of proteins was suspended in PBS and matrix metalloproteinase-8 (MMP-8) concentration was determined by Immunoplex assay (Millipore, Burlington, MA, USA) using Bioplex instrument [25].

2.6. Statistical Analysis

For continuous variables, multiple group comparisons were performed by the Kruskal–Wallis test, while for two-group comparisons the Mann–Whitney U test was used. Spearman's rank correlation test was used to examine the relationships between two continuous variables. Analysis of covariance (ANCOVA) was applied to compare cervix length among CSTs, obstetric diseases, and gestational diabetes mellitus groups, adjusting for gestational age at sampling or for age of patients. For the analysis of frequency, statistical analyses were performed using Fisher's exact test. For each odds ratio, a confidence interval at 95% (CI 95%) was shown, and the z test was applied to obtain a p-value associated with OR. $p < 0.05$ was considered significant. Statistical analysis was performed using R software version 4.0.2.

3. Results

3.1. Population

During the study period, 174 potential study participants who met the inclusion criteria were identified. Of these, 128 were excluded because they presented one or more of the exclusion criteria. Therefore, 46 women were enrolled in the study. Table 1 summarizes demographic and clinical information of the enrolled patients, including age (34.2 ± 6.7 years; mean ± SD), gestational age (GA) at sampling (27.6 ± 2; mean ± SD), and pregnancy complications including GDM (diagnosed in 10/46 pregnant women, and requiring insulin treatment in 5 of them). GDM was diagnosed using the 2 h 75 g oral glucose tolerance test at 24 to 28 weeks' gestation, or earlier in patients at high risk for gestational diabetes. The mean gestational age at diagnosis was 25.1 weeks. Vaginal infections that occurred later in gestation were also reported. In our cohort of women, those enrolled at 28 to 32 weeks all had a cervical length <20 mm and 38% of them had a cervical length <10 mm. Progesterone therapy was administered to all women after sample collection to reduce the risk of sPTB throughout gestation. Overall, 10 women (21.7%) delivered preterm (<37 weeks' gestation): of these, three belonged to the group with extreme cervical shortening (<11 mm), six to the group with cervical length 11–20 mm, and only one to the group with cervical length 21–24 mm. The relationship between specific CSTs and PTB was not analyzed, as the study was not powered to evaluate this outcome.

Table 1. Patient demographic and clinical information.

	All Women, n (%)	Stratification by Cervical Length (<25 mm)			p-Value (Chi Square Test)
		1–10 mm	11–20 mm	21–24 mm	
N. of enrolled women at risk of sPTB	46 (100%)	15 (32.6%)	25 (54.3%)	6 (13%)	
Ethnicity					
Caucasian	44 (95.7%)	15 (100%)	23 (92%)	6 (100%)	
Asian	1 (2.2%)	0 (0%)	1 (4%)	0 (0%)	
North-African (Morocco)	1 (2.2%)	0 (0%)	1 (4%)	0 (0%)	
Age at sampling (years); mean ± SD	34.2 ± 6.7	34.1 ± 6.5	34.7 ± 7.1	32.2 ± 6.4	
Gestational age at sampling (weeks); mean ± SD	27.6 ± 2	27.9 ± 2.2	27.6 ± 2.1	26.8 ± 1.5	
Pregnancy complications					
Vaginal infection [1]	11 (23.9%)	5 (33.3%)	4 (16%)	1 (16.6%)	0.415
GDM	10 (21.7%)	1 (6.66%)	7 (28%)	2 (33.3%)	0.217

[1] Vaginal infections included yeast infection and bacterial vaginosis (such as *Streptococcus*, *Gardnerella*, *Ureaplasma*, *Klebsiella* and *Citrobacter*). These infections were diagnosed at a later gestational age than enrolment and sample collection, when the patient reported vaginal symptoms. sPTB, Spontaneous preterm birth; GDM, gestational diabetes mellitus

As the first step of our analysis, we evaluated whether maternal age and/or the presence of GDM can affect cervical shortening. Supplementary Figure S1A shows that there were no significant differences in cervical length between women with GDM and women who did not develop GDM. Similarly, no significant correlations between GA at sampling or maternal age and cervical length were detected (Supplementary Figure S1B,C).

3.2. Vaginal Microbiota Composition

The vaginal samples were first classified into two categories based on *Lactobacillus* abundance (Figure 1A): (i) *Lactobacillus*-dominated (≥50% *Lactobacillus* spp.); and (ii) Lactobacillus-depleted microbiota (<10% *Lactobacillus* spp.). The *Lactobacillus*-dominated microbiota category was the most prevalent in our cohort (n = 40; 86.9%), while the *Lactobacillus*-depleted microbiota was only present in 6 women (13%). Spearman correlation analysis showed that the abundance of taxa belonging to the *Lactobacillus* genus was positively correlated with cervical length (Spearman coefficient 0.421; $p = 0.01$). Figure 1B shows that women with *Lactobacillus*-depleted microbiota had an extremely short cervix length (<10 mm) and significant differences were recorded by comparing the cervical length of these women with that of women with *Lactobacillus*-dominated microbiota. When the cervical length of these two groups was adjusted for maternal age or GA, no interaction between grouping variable (*Lactobacillus*-depleted/-dominated microbiota) and covariates was found by ANCOVA analysis (Supplementary Table S1 and Figure S2), supporting the significance of differences in cervical length between women with *Lactobacillus*-depleted microbiota and women with *Lactobacillus*-dominated microbiota (Figure 1C,D).

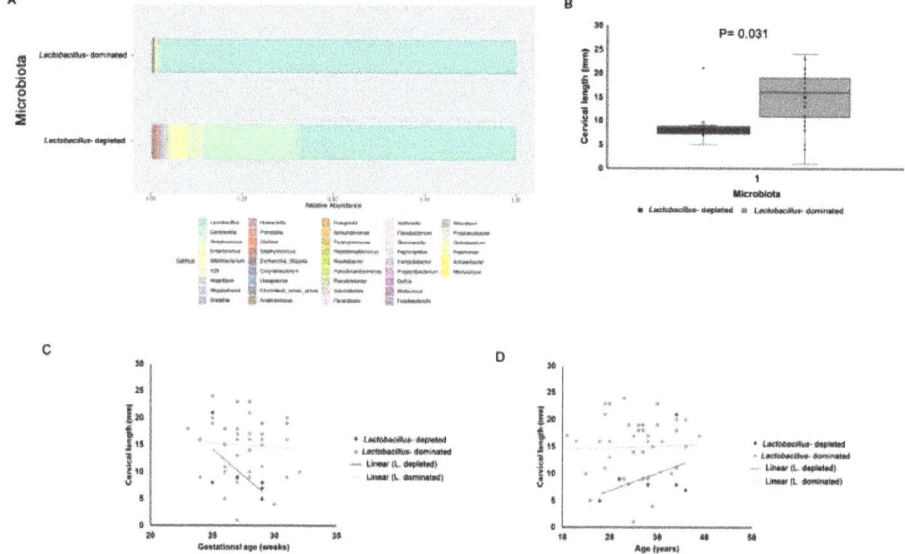

Figure 1. Survey of vaginal microbiota and correlation with cervical length. (**A**) Overview of vaginal microbiota grouped by *Lactobacillus*-depleted and *Lactobacillus*-dominated microbiota types. In each barplot, the percentage of relative abundances at the genus level is showed. (**B**) Differences in cervical length between women with *Lactobacillus*-depleted microbiota and women with *Lactobacillus*-dominated microbiota. Data are presented as box and whisker plots, with boxes extending from the 25th to 75th percentile and horizontal lines representing the median. Whiskers extend 1.5 times the interquartile range from the 25th and 75th percentile. Statistical analysis was performed by Mann–Whitney assay. *p*-value < 0.05 was considered as significant. (**C,D**) Analysis of covariance (ANCOVA) with grouping variables and covariates (**C**) age and (**D**) gestational age at sampling. Scatter plot with regression lines for the two groups (*Lactobacillus*-depleted/*Lactobacillus*-dominated microbiota).

3.3. Community State Type (CST) Distribution of Vaginal Microbiota

To deeper understand vaginal microbiota composition and to define microbial profiles associated with extreme cervical shortening, we stratified vaginal microbiotas into the five major vaginal community state types (CSTs), according to Ravel J et al. [11].

L. crispatus-dominated microbiota (CST-I) characterized 34.8% ($n = 16$) of pregnant women, *L. gasseri*-dominated microbiota (CST-II) was present in 13% ($n = 6$), *L. iners*-dominated microbiota (CST-III) in 32.6% ($n = 15$), *L. jensenii*-dominated microbiota (CST-V) in 6.5% ($n = 3$) of women (Table 2). *Lactobacillus*-depleted microbiota, defined as CST-IV was found in 13% ($n = 6$) of our patients (Table 2).

Fisher's Exact test showed a statistically significant difference in the distribution of CSTs in women with different cervical length ($p = 0.007$; Table 2).

Table 2. Distribution of CSTs in all recruited women, according to cervical length. We differentiated the women with a very short cervix (1–10 mm) from the others (11–24 mm).

	All Women	Cervical Length		p-Value (Fisher's Exact Test)
		1–10 mm	11–24 mm	
Total N	46	15	31	
CST I	16 (34.8%)	3 (20.0%)	13 (41.9%)	
CST II	6 (13.0%)	0 (0.0%)	6 (19.4%)	0.007
CST III	15 (32.6%)	7 (46.7%)	8 (25.8%)	
CST IV	6 (13.0%)	5 (33.3%)	1 (3.2%)	
CST V	2 (6.5%)	0 (0.0%)	3 (9.7%)	

To evaluate the distribution of cervical samples based on their microbial community composition, we performed PCoA ordination based on Bray-Curtis distances (Figure 2). This analysis showed that the distribution of the vaginal samples was clearly driven by CSTs (PERMANOVA, $p = 0.001$).

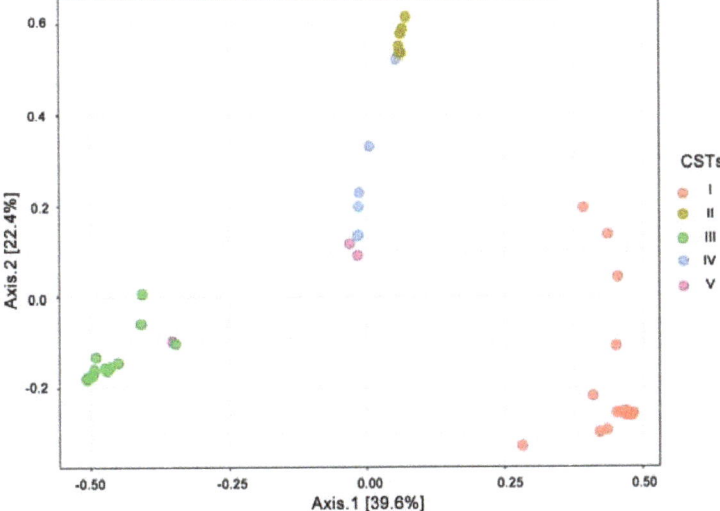

Figure 2. Beta diversity measure. Principal Coordinate Analysis (PCoA) ordination based on Bray Curtis dissimilarities correlated with community state types (CSTs) (permutational multivariate analysis of variance (PERMANOVA) 999 permutations; $R2 = 0.740$ p-value < 0.001). Samples belonging to different CSTs are indicated with different colour dots.

Moreover, the differential abundance of *Lactobacillus* and *Gardnerella* genera reflected the distribution among samples (Supplementary Figure S3; PERMANOVA $R2 = 0.741$; $p < 0.001$). PERMANOVA analysis showed that no other variables, such as cervical length, or the presence of GDM, differed between CST types (Supplementary Table S2).

In accordance with the data shown in Figure 1B, OR calculation showed that vaginal microbiota of CST-IV type was the main risk factor for extreme cervical shortening (OR = 15 CI = 1.56–144.0; $p = 0.019$).

However, due to the high prevalence of women of Caucasian ethnicity in our cohort, CST-IV was present in only 13% of vaginal swabs, while *Lactobacillus*-dominated CSTs were largely represented in 87% of samples (Table 2). Thus, we decided to analyse only the *Lactobacillus*-dominated vaginal microbiota samples. We observed that in 7/15 women (46.7%) with an extremely short cervix (1–10 mm) the vaginal community was dominated by *L. iners* (Table 2). Statistical analyses indeed showed that, among *Lactobacillus*-dominated CSTs (CST I, CST II, CST III, CST V), women with CST III microbiota had the highest risk of having an extremely short cervix (OR = 6.4 CI 95% = 1.32–31.032; *p*-value = 0.024; Table 3). This suggests that CST-III might be the only community among that *Lactobacillus* dominated-species possibly involved in the mechanisms leading to severe cervical shortening.

Table 3. Association of CSTs and cervical shortening categorization.

Vaginal Microbial Community	Cervical Length		*p*-Value (Fisher's Exact Test)	OR	95% CI	*p*-Value OR
	1–10 mm	11–24 mm				
L. iners-dominated community (CST III)	7 (46.7%)	8 (25.8%)	0.191	2.52	0.69–9.18	0.16
other CSTs	8 (53.3%)	23 (74.2%)				
L. iners-dominated community (CST III)	7 (70.0%)	8 (26.7%)	0.024	6.417	1.327–31.032	0.021
other *Lactobacillus* spp.-dominated community (CST I, CST II, CST V)	3 (30.0%)	22 (73.3%)				

We also measured MMP-8 concentration in supernatant of cervical samples, since this enzyme is known to compromise the epithelial barrier integrity [26] and was found to be strongly associated with cervical shortening [27]. We found an increased concentration of MMP-8 in women with CST III and CST IV microbiota compared to other CSTs groups (*Lactobacillus*-dominated community; CST I, CST II, and CST V). The difference, however, did not reach statistical significance (Supplementary Figure S4).

3.4. Cervical Shortening, Microbial Diversity and Enrichment of Bacterial Taxa

When pregnant women were stratified in three subgroups based on cervical shortening (1–10 mm, 11–20 mm, 21–24 mm), microbial diversity seemed to increase with progressive cervical shortening, as shown by barplot configuration of microbiota composition in vaginal samples (Figure 3A). We used these groups of samples to further identify differential microbial profiles associated with cervical shortening. In particular, a progressive reduction of *Lactobacillus* spp. and an increase of *Gardnerella*, *Streptococcus*, *Enterococcus* and *Prevotella* genera were evident in groups with the shortest cervix (Figure 3A). Estimation of species richness (alpha diversity) was also measured (Supplementary Figure S5). Although a trend toward an increased microbial diversity was evident in the 1–10 mm and 11–20 mm groups compared to the 21–24 mm group, no statistically significant differences in species richness were observed by ANOVA analysis.

The enrichment of selected bacterial taxa in groups of women with different cervical length was evaluated by LEfSe. By pairwise comparison of vaginal samples of women with cervical length 1–10 mm versus 21–24 mm (Figure 3B), we confirmed enrichment of *Lactobacillus* spp. in women with cervical length approaching the limit of 25 mm (21–24 mm). Taxa from the *Bifidobacteriaceae* family and, in particular, *Gardnerella* genus were enriched in women with a cervical length ranging from 11 to 20 mm, compared with women with a cervical length of 21–24 mm (Figure 3C). LEfSe, however, did not show discriminative bacterial profiles when samples of women with cervical length between 1 and 10 mm were compared to those of women with cervical length between 11 and 20 mm.

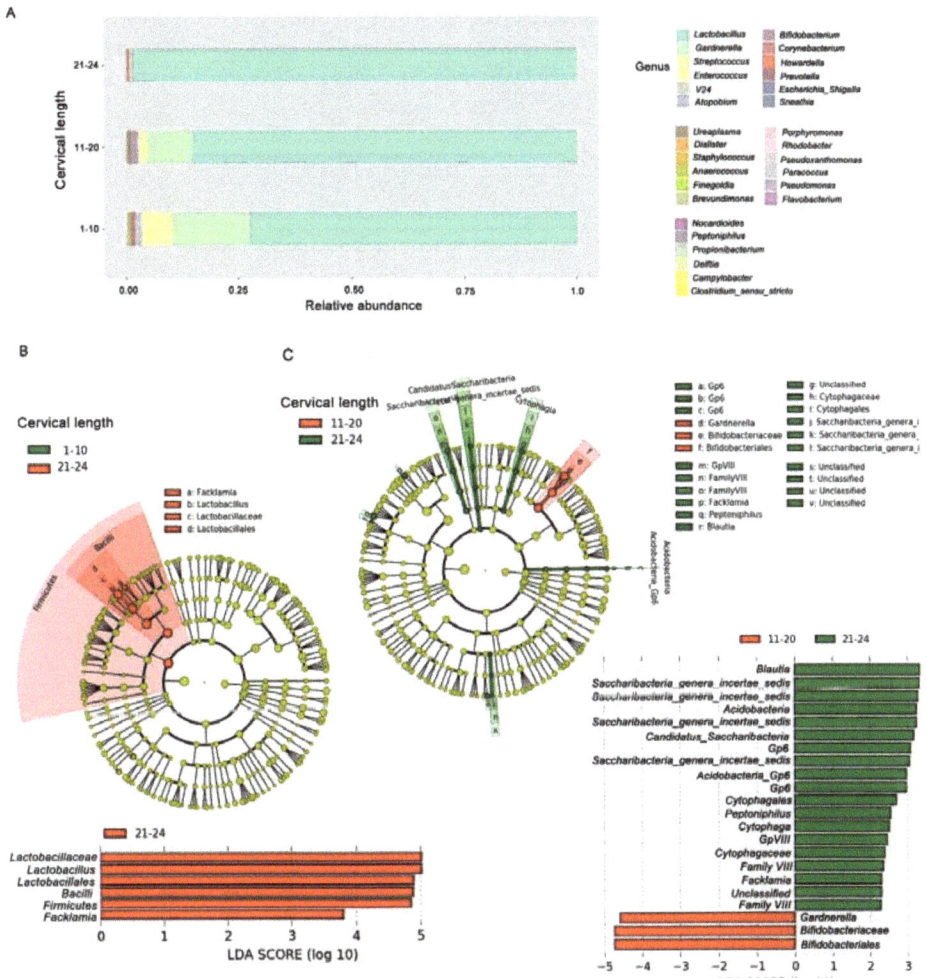

Figure 3. Microbiome profiles in vaginal samples according to cervical shortening categorization. (**A**) Barplot of vaginal swab samples was stratified based on cervical shortening (1–10 mm, 11–20 mm, 21–24 mm). The percentage of bacterial relative abundances (average) at the genus level is showed. (**B**,**C**) Metagenomic biomarker discovery by linear discriminant analysis effect size (LEfSe) analysis. Comparison of enriched taxa between vaginal samples of women with cervix length (**B**) 1–10 mm vs. 21–24 mm, and (**C**) 11–20 mm vs. 21–24 mm. Results indicated the statistically significant taxa enrichment among groups (Alpha value = 0.05 for the factorial Kruskal–Wallis test among classes). The threshold for the logarithmic LDA score was 2.0.

3.5. Gestational Diabetes Mellitus, Vaginal Microbiota Profile and Cervical Shortening

In our cohort, 21.7% (10/46) of pregnant women were diagnosed with GDM (Table 1), a metabolic disorder that may affect the composition of the vaginal microbiota [19]. CSTs distribution of microbiota from women with GDM revealed 3 CST-I, 3 CST-III, 3 CST IV, and 1 CST-V. No difference in the distribution of samples based on GDM was highlighted by the PCoA ordination (PERMANOVA; Supplementary Table S2). Moreover, as indicated above, Figure 1A shows no statistically significant differences in the cervical length between women with GDM and those not affected.

Although the number of women with GDM was limited, we noted that alpha diversity indexes (observed OTUs and Chao I) were significantly higher in women experiencing GDM compared with non-diabetic women (Figure 4A).

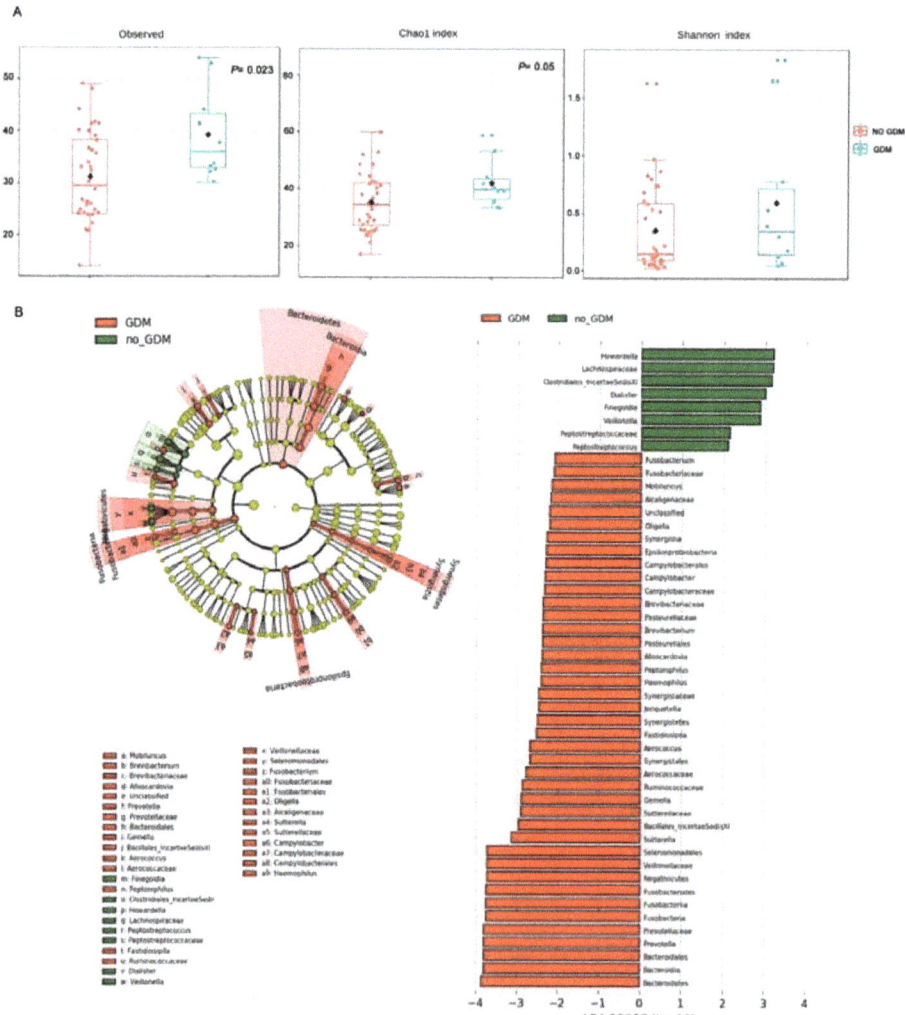

Figure 4. Vaginal microbiome profiles of women experiencing GDM during the pregnancy. (**A**) Alpha diversity (observed operational taxonomic units (OTUs), Chao I and Shannon indexes; *p*-values by Kruskal–Wallis test). (**B**) LEfSe analysis. Comparison of enriched taxa between vaginal samples of women with GDM and normal glucose-tolerant women. Results indicated the statistically significant taxa enrichment among groups (Alpha value = 0.05 for the factorial Kruskal–Wallis test among classes). The threshold for the logarithmic LDA score was 2.0.

To investigate the reasons for this increase in bacterial richness in more depth, we compared vaginal microbial profiles of women experiencing GDM during pregnancy with those of non-diabetic women. LEfSe analysis revealed significant enrichment of taxa in association with GDM, such as *Fusobacterium, Mobiluncus, Prevotella, Brevibacterium*, and taxa from the families of *Enterobacteriaceae* (*Campylobacter, Haemophilus*), *Aerococcaceae, Sutterellaceae* and *Lachnospiraceae* (Figure 4B). When women with GDM were considered as a subclass stratified based on cervical shortening, LEfSe analysis did not reveal significant enrichment of bacterial taxa, indicating no association between specific microbiota profiles and short cervix in women with GDM.

4. Discussion

In our study, microbiota analysis of vaginal fluids was performed in a selected cohort of pregnant women with cervical shortening during the second or early third trimester of pregnancy, to identify vaginal communities associated with "extreme" cervical shortening (1–10 mm), a high-risk factor for spontaneous preterm birth [1–3]. A cervical length shorter than 10 mm is considered abnormal (below the 5th or 10th percentile for gestational age) even at 28–32 weeks' gestation [1,20]. Iams et al. [1] reported that the relative risk of PTB increased as the length of the cervix decreased: they observed that the RR for PTB was 9.49 (95% CI 5.95–15.15) for lengths at or below the 5th percentile at 24 weeks (22 mm), and 13.99 (95% CI 7.89 to 24.78) for lengths at or below the 1st percentile (13 mm), compared with those above the 75th percentile. At 28 weeks, the corresponding relative risks for preterm delivery were 13.88 and 24.94.

In agreement with Gerson et al. [8], we found that *Lactobacillus*-abundance was positively correlated with cervical length. In contrast, *Lactobacillus*-depleted communities, which define the microbiota commonly named CST-IV [11], were significantly associated with increased odds of extreme cervical shortening (OR = 15 CI = 1.56–144; p = 0.019). Taking into account the higher stability of vaginal microbiota during pregnancy compared to non-pregnant status [17], these data reinforce the concept that *Lactobacillus*-depleted communities leading to vaginal dysbiosis are a risk factor for cervical insufficiency and remodeling of the cervix during pregnancy. *Lactobacillus*-dominated communities of the vagina are known to inhibit the adhesion and proliferation of opportunistic and primary pathogens [28] through multiple mechanisms including the production of antimicrobial compounds, such as hydrogen peroxide, lactic acid and/or bacteriocins, acting as a biosurfactant on the vaginal epithelium [10].

The occurrence of communities with low proportions or no detectable *Lactobacillus* spp. are relatively uncommon in the vaginal environment of non-pregnant white Caucasian women (10.3%) or Asian women (19.8%) compared with Hispanic (38.1%) and Black (40.4%) women [11].

In our cohort, white Caucasian women represented 96% of cases, Asian 2.1%, and only one woman was from North-Africa (Arabian ethnicity). *Lactobacillus*-dominated communities were present in 86% of vaginal swabs. Although our data confirmed the association between CST-IV and extremely short cervix [8], we also evaluated whether other microbial communities, more represented in white Caucasian women, could also be associated with the risk of an extremely short cervix. Our results showed that about half of women with *L. iners*-dominated communities (CST-III) had an extremely short cervix at the time of sampling, suggesting that *L. iners* may play a role in the mechanisms of cervical shortening and remodeling during pregnancy. Compared to the other species of Lactobacilli evolutionary adapted in the vaginal environment, *L. iners* is the species with the lowest ability to contrast infections from external pathogens or pathobionts. *L. iners* produces D-lactate instead of L-lactate, low amounts of antimicrobial peptides, and has reduced ability to bind epithelial cells [12]. For these reasons, *L. iners* has reduced ability to prevent the enrichment of *Gardnerella* and other bacteria causing bacterial vaginosis and it is better adapted to vaginal dysbiosis-associated conditions, such as an elevated pH and the presence of polymicrobial communities [10,12,29,30].

L. iners has been suggested as a marker of microbial imbalance leading to bacterial vaginosis [31]. Moreover, it was reported that *L. iners* increases ectocervical and endocervical permeability, suggesting that this bacterial species is less active in modulating inflammatory processes that could have negative consequences on cervical length during pregnancy [31].

Kindinger et al. [32] found a significant positive association between *L. iners*-dominated communities (CST-III) and the occurrence of spontaneous pre-term birth in a cohort of predominantly Caucasian and Asian women. In our study, the *L. iners*-dominated community was the only *Lactobacillus*-enriched community significantly associated with an extremely short cervix (1–10 mm; OR = 6.4; p = 0.02) suggesting that, besides CST-IV, CST-III may serve as a marker of increased risk of extreme cervical shortening, in particular in women of Caucasian ethnicity.

Finally, it is known that insulin resistance, weight gain and increased inflammation in women developing GDM may play a role in favoring adaptation of microbial communities that are different from those of non-diabetic women [19]. An abundance of potentially pathogenic bacteria and an increase of inflammatory cytokines expression have been described in the vaginal microbiome of women with GDM. We thus investigated whether, in our cohort, women experiencing GDM during pregnancy have a different vaginal microbial profile compared to women who did not develop GDM. In accordance with Cortez et al. [19], we found that the vaginal microbial profiles of women with GDM were enriched of bacterial taxa abundant in vaginal dysbiosis or associated with a viral infection, inflammation or epithelial adhesiveness [13,33] compared to non-diabetic women. Despite these results, we could not associate GDM with extreme cervical shortening. Further studies in a larger cohort of pregnant women are needed to define whether GDM or other complications during the pregnancy are involved in the mechanism leading to cervical shortening.

Strengths of the present study include the cross-sectional design and the selection of a group of mostly Caucasian women, who generally have a vaginal microbiota enriched with *Lactobacillus* spp. compared to other ethnicities, to investigate the association between microbial profiles/CSTs and a shortened cervical length. Furthermore, vaginal sampling was performed before any mitigative or therapeutic measures in order to limit the amount of confounding factors.

This study presents some limitations: (i) only one sample of vaginal fluid was collected from each woman for vaginal microbiota investigation. This may represent a limitation, as it does not allow for evaluating the dynamics of the microbiota with progressive cervical shortening during pregnancy. However, some evidence indicated that, during physiologic pregnancy, vaginal microbiota is more stable compared to non-pregnant women [18]; (ii) assessing the global vaginal microbiota community by 16S rRNA gene-based amplicon sequencing limits the evaluation of every single bacterial contribution to the mechanisms leading to cervical shortening; (iii) we could not draw any conclusion on the relationship between specific CSTs and PTB, as the study was not powered to evaluate this outcome. Moreover, the treatment of most women with progesterone therapy limited the ability to evaluate such association; (iv) the study did not include a control group of women with cervical length >25 mm, which would have allowed comparison of microbial profiles according to cervical length; (v): the exclusion of patients who had a pessary placed for prevention of PTB could represent a selection bias. At the time of the study at our institution, the cervical pessary was placed, with specific indications, during hospital admission and then the patients received follow-up at our preterm birth clinic. Therefore, we did not include this subset of patients, as the impact that the pessary might have on the vaginal microbiota is not well known.

This study showed that CST-IV is a risk factor for extreme cervical shortening in Caucasian women. *L. iners*-dominated community (CST III), a type of vaginal microbiota much more common in white Caucasian women, was identified as an additional risk factor for extreme cervical shortening. Future studies exploring the microbial contribution to the mechanisms leading to severe cervical shortening will be crucial in predicting susceptibility to sPTB.

Supplementary Materials: The following are available online at http://www.mdpi.com/2077-0383/9/11/3621/s1, Figure S1: (a) Differences in cervical length (mm) between patients with or without GDM. Statistical analysis was performed by the Mann–Whitney test, p-value = 0.161. (b) The relationship between cervical length (mm) and gestational age (weeks) was investigated by the Spearman's rank correlation test. No statistically significant correlation was found (Spearman's rank correlation coefficient −0.108, p value = 0.475). (c) The relationship between cervical length (mm) and age (years) was investigated by Spearman's rank correlation test. No statistically significant correlation was found (Spearman's rank correlation coefficient 0.0451, p-value = 0.766). Figure S2: Subgroups examination and ANCOVA analysis. (a) The ANCOVA analysis shows that no differences in cervical length between women with or without gestational diabetes mellitus were found when the data were adjusted for gestational age at sampling (p-value 0.308). The same analysis shows that no correlation exists between gestational age and cervical length in each subgroup considered. In addition, the ANCOVA analysis revealed that no interaction between the covariate (gestational age at sampling) and grouping variables (gestational diabetes mellitus) exist (p-value 0.851). Left panel: scatter plot with regression lines for the two groups (diabetes mellitus yes or no); right panel: output from R software version 4.0.2 for ANCOVA analysis. (b) The ANCOVA analysis shows that no differences in cervical length between women with or without gestational diabetes mellitus were found when the data were adjusted for gestational age at sampling (p-value 0.253). The same analysis shows that no correlation exists between gestational age and cervix length in each subgroup considered. In addition, the ANCOVA analysis revealed that no interaction between the covariate (gestational age at sampling) and grouping variables (gestational diabetes mellitus) exist (p-value 0.741). Left panel: scatter plot with regression lines for the two groups (diabetes mellitus yes or no); right panel: output from R software version 4.0.2 for ANCOVA analysis. Figure S3: PCoA ordination, based on Bray Curtis dissimilarities, correlated with (a) *Lactobacillus* spp. and (b) *Gardnerella* spp. abundances. Colors from red to green indicate a decreasing abundance of the bacterial genus (PERMANOVA 999 permutations; R20.740 p-value < 0.001). Figure S4: Matrix metalloprotease 8 (MMP-8) concentration in vaginal samples of a subgroup of women. Data from pregnant women with vaginal microbiota of CST-I, CST-II, and CST-V (*Lactobacillus*-dominated community) were compared with data from women with CST-III (*L. iners*-dominated) and CST-IV (*Lactobacillus*-depleted). Data are presented as box and whisker plots, with boxes extending from the 25th to 75th percentile and horizontal lines representing the median. Whiskers extend 1.5 times the interquartile range from the 25th and 75th percentile. Statistical analysis, performed by the Mann–Whitney assay did not reveal significant differences. Figure S5: Alpha diversity measures. Box plots of observed OTUs, Chao 1, and Shannon index according to the cervical length classification. ANOVA test resulted not significant for all comparisons. Table S1: ANCOVA analysis with microbiota as a grouping variable and gestational age at sampling as covariate adjustment. The output from R software version 4.0.2 for ANCOVA analysis. Table S2: PERMANOVA analysis on PCoA ordination of vaginal microbiota samples.

Author Contributions: Conceptualization, M.D.T., M.G.T., A.P. and C.D.F.; methodology, M.D.P., V.S., S.P.; formal analysis M.D.P., C.L., M.T., F.V.; investigation, M.D.P., V.S., A.P., C.D.F., M.D.T.; writing—original draft preparation, M.D.P., V.S., M.G.T.; funding acquisition, M.D.T. and M.G.T. All authors have read and agreed to the published version of the manuscript.

Funding: This research was funded by Ente Cassa di Risparmio di Firenze, 2016 and by Project V.A.M.P., Regione Toscana 2018.

Acknowledgments: The authors wish to thank all patients who donated biological material for the purposes of the study and are very grateful to Steven S. Witkin for critical reading of the manuscript and his useful suggestions.

Conflicts of Interest: The authors declare no conflict of interest.

References

1. Iams, J.D.; Goldenberg, R.L.; Meis, P.J.; Mercer, B.M.; Moawad, A.; Das, A.; Thom, E.; McNellis, D.; Copper, R.L.; Johnson, F.; et al. The length of the cervix and the risk of spontaneous premature delivery. *N. Engl. J. Med.* **1996**, *334*, 567–572. [CrossRef]
2. Di Tommaso, M.; Berghella, V. Cervical length for the prediction and prevention of preterm birth. *Expert Rev. Obstet. Gynecol.* **2013**, *8*, 345–355. [CrossRef]
3. Goldenberg, R.L.; Andrews, W.; Guerrant, R.; Newman, M.; Mercer, B.; Iams, J.; Meis, P.; Moawad, A.; Das, A.; VanDorsten, J.; et al. The preterm prediction study: Cervical lactoferrin concentration, other markers of lower genital tract infection, and preterm birth. *Am. J. Obstet. Gynecol.* **2000**, *182*, 631–635. [CrossRef] [PubMed]
4. Owen, J.; Yost, N.; Berghella, V.; Thom, E.; Swain, M.; Iii, G.A.D.; Miodovnik, M.; Langer, O.; Sibai, B.; McNellis, D.; et al. Mid-trimester endovaginal sonography in women at high risk for spontaneous preterm birth. *JAMA* **2001**, *286*, 1340–1348. [CrossRef] [PubMed]
5. Singer, M.S.; Hochman, M. Incompetent cervix in a hormone-exposed offspring. *Obstet. Gynecol.* **1978**, *51*, 625–626. [CrossRef]
6. Hordnes, K. Ehlers-Danlos syndrome and delivery. *Acta Obstet. Gynecol. Scand.* **1994**, *73*, 671–673. [CrossRef]
7. Check, J.H.; Lee, G.; Epstein, R.; Vetter, B. Increased rate of preterm deliveries in untreated women with luteal phase deficiencies. Preliminary report. *Gynecol. Obstet. Investig.* **1992**, *33*, 183–184. [CrossRef]
8. Gerson, K.D.; McCarthy, C.; Elovitz, M.A.; Ravel, J.; Sammel, M.D.; Burris, H.H. Cervicovaginal microbial communities deficient in Lactobacillus species are associated with second trimester short cervix. *Am. J. Obstet. Gynecol.* **2020**, *222*, 491.e1–491.e8. [CrossRef]

9. Kroon, S.J.; Ravel, J.; Huston, W.M. Cervicovaginal microbiota, women's health, and reproductive outcomes. *Fertil. Steril.* **2018**, *110*, 327–336. [CrossRef]
10. Aldunate, M.; Srbinovski, D.; Hearps, A.C.; Latham, C.F.; Ramsland, P.A.; Gugasyan, R.; Cone, R.A.; Tachedjian, G. Antimicrobial and immune modulatory effects of lactic acid and short chain fatty acids produced by vaginal microbiota associated with eubiosis and bacterial vaginosis. *Front. Physiol.* **2015**, *6*, 164. [CrossRef]
11. Ravel, J.; Gajer, P.; Abdo, Z.; Schneider, G.M.; Koenig, S.S.K.; McCulle, S.L.; Karlebach, S.; Gorle, R.; Russell, J.; Tacket, C.O.; et al. Vaginal microbiome of reproductive-age women. *Proc. Natl. Acad. Sci. USA* **2011**, *108* (Suppl. 1), 4680–4687. [CrossRef] [PubMed]
12. Torcia, M.G. Interplay among Vaginal Microbiome, Immune Response and Sexually Transmitted Viral Infections. *Int. J. Mol. Sci.* **2019**, *20*, 266. [CrossRef] [PubMed]
13. Di Paola, M.; Sani, C.; Clemente, A.M.; Iossa, A.; Perissi, E.; Castronovo, G.; Tanturli, M.; Rivero, D.; Cozzolino, F.; Cavalieri, D.; et al. Characterization of cervico-vaginal microbiota in women developing persistent high-risk Human Papillomavirus infection. *Sci. Rep.* **2017**, *7*, 10200. [CrossRef] [PubMed]
14. Onywera, H.; Williamson, A.L.; Mbulawa, Z.Z.A.; Coetzee, D.; Meiring, T.L. Factors associated with the composition and diversity of the cervical microbiota of reproductive-age Black South African women: A retrospective cross-sectional study. *PeerJ* **2019**, *7*, e7488. [CrossRef] [PubMed]
15. Laniewski, P.; Barnes, D.; Goulder, A.; Cui, H.; Roe, D.J.; Chase, D.M.; Herbst-Kralovetz, M.M. Linking cervicovaginal immune signatures, HPV and microbiota composition in cervical carcinogenesis in non-Hispanic and Hispanic women. *Sci. Rep.* **2018**, *8*, 7593. [CrossRef]
16. Aagaard, K.; Riehle, K.; Ma, J.; Segata, N.; Mistretta, T.-A.; Coarfa, C.; Raza, S.; Rosenbaum, S.; Veyver, I.V.D.; Milosavljevic, A.; et al. A metagenomic approach to characterization of the vaginal microbiome signature in pregnancy. *PLoS ONE* **2012**, *7*, e36466. [CrossRef]
17. Romero, R.; Hassan, S.S.; Gajer, P.; Tarca, A.L.; Fadrosh, D.W.; Nikita, L.; Galuppi, M.; Lamont, R.F.; Chaemsaithong, P.; Miranda, J.; et al. The composition and stability of the vaginal microbiota of normal pregnant women is different from that of non-pregnant women. *Microbiome* **2014**, *2*, 4. [CrossRef]
18. Witkin, S.S.; Moron, A.F.; Ridenhour, B.J.; Minis, E.; Hatanaka, A.; Sarmento, S.G.P.; Franca, M.S.; Carvalho, F.H.C.; Hamamoto, T.K.; Mattar, R.; et al. Vaginal Biomarkers That Predict Cervical Length and Dominant Bacteria in the Vaginal Microbiomes of Pregnant Women. *mBio.* **2019**, *10*, e02242-19. [CrossRef]
19. Cortez, R.V.; Taddei, C.R.; Sparvoli, L.G.; Angelo, A.G.S.; Padilha, M.; Mattar, R.; Daher, S. Microbiome and its relation to gestational diabetes. *Endocrine* **2019**, *64*, 254–264. [CrossRef]
20. Berghella, V.; Roman, A.; Daskalakis, C.; Ness, A.; Baxter, J.K. Gestational age at cervical length measurement and incidence of preterm birth. *Obstet. Gynecol.* **2007**, *2 Pt 1*, 311–317. [CrossRef]
21. Albanese, D.; Fontana, P.; De Filippo, C.; Cavalieri, D.; Donati, C. MICCA: A complete and accurate software for taxonomic profiling of metagenomic data. *Sci. Rep.* **2015**, *5*, 9743. [CrossRef] [PubMed]
22. Meriggi, N.; Di Paola, M.; Vitali, F.; Rivero, D.; Cappa, F.; Turillazzi, F.; Gori, A.; Dapporto, L.; Beani, L.; Turillazzi, S.; et al. Saccharomyces cerevisiae Induces Immune Enhancing and Shapes Gut Microbiota in Social Wasps. *Front. Microbiol.* **2019**, *10*, 2320. [CrossRef] [PubMed]
23. McMurdie, P.J.; Holmes, S. phyloseq: An R package for reproducible interactive analysis and graphics of microbiome census data. *PLoS ONE* **2013**, *8*, e61217. [CrossRef] [PubMed]
24. Dhariwal, A.; Chong, J.; Habib, S.; King, I.L.; Agellon, L.B.; Xia, J. MicrobiomeAnalyst: A web-based tool for comprehensive statistical, visual and meta-analysis of microbiome data. *Nucleic Acids Res.* **2017**, *45*, W180–W188. [CrossRef] [PubMed]
25. Celestino, I.; Checconi, P.; Amatore, D.; De Angelis, M.; Coluccio, P.; Dattilo, R.; Fegatelli, D.A.; Clemente, A.M.; Matarrese, P.; Torcia, M.G.; et al. Differential Redox State Contributes to Sex Disparities in the Response to Influenza Virus Infection in Male and Female Mice. *Front. Immunol.* **2018**, *9*, 1747. [CrossRef] [PubMed]
26. Van Lint, P.; Libert, C. Matrix metalloproteinase-8: Cleavage can be decisive. *Cytokine Growth Factor Rev.* **2006**, *17*, 217–223. [CrossRef]
27. Sisti, G.; Paccosi, S.; Parenti, A.; Seravalli, V.; Linari, C.; Di Tommaso, M.; Witkin, S. Pro-inflammatory mediators in vaginal fluid and short cervical length in pregnancy. *Bratisl. Lek. Listy* **2020**, *121*, 278–281.
28. Bolton, M.; van der Straten, A.; Cohen, C.R. Probiotics: Potential to prevent HIV and sexually transmitted infections in women. *Sex. Transm. Dis.* **2008**, *35*, 214–225. [CrossRef]

29. Peelen, M.J.; Luef, B.M.; Lamont, R.F.; De Milliano, I.; Jensen, J.S.; Limpens, J.; Hajenius, P.J.; Jørgensen, J.S.; Menon, R. The influence of the vaginal microbiota on preterm birth: A systematic review and recommendations for a minimum dataset for future research. *Placenta* **2019**, *79*, 30–39. [CrossRef]
30. Amabebe, E.; Anumba, D.O.C. The Vaginal Microenvironment: The Physiologic Role of Lactobacilli. *Front. Med.* **2018**, *5*, 181. [CrossRef]
31. Africa, C.W.; Nel, J.; Stemmet, M. Anaerobes and bacterial vaginosis in pregnancy: Virulence factors contributing to vaginal colonisation. *Int. J. Environ. Res. Public Health* **2014**, *11*, 6979–7000. [CrossRef] [PubMed]
32. Kindinger, L.M.; Bennett, P.R.; Lee, Y.S.; Marchesi, J.R.; Smith, A.; Cacciatore, S.; Holmes, E.; Nicholson, J.K.; Teoh, T.G.; MacIntyre, D.A. The interaction between vaginal microbiota, cervical length, and vaginal progesterone treatment for preterm birth risk. *Microbiome* **2017**, *5*, 6. [CrossRef] [PubMed]
33. Galaz, J.; Romero, R.; Slutsky, R.; Xu, Y.; Motomura, K.; Para, R.; Pacora, P.; Panaitescu, B.; Hsu, C.-D.; Kacerovsky, M.; et al. Cellular immune responses in amniotic fluid of women with preterm prelabor rupture of membranes. *J. Perinat. Med.* **2020**, *48*, 222–233. [CrossRef] [PubMed]

Publisher's Note: MDPI stays neutral with regard to jurisdictional claims in published maps and institutional affiliations.

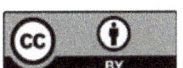

© 2020 by the authors. Licensee MDPI, Basel, Switzerland. This article is an open access article distributed under the terms and conditions of the Creative Commons Attribution (CC BY) license (http://creativecommons.org/licenses/by/4.0/).

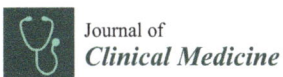

Review

Prevention of Preterm Birth with Progesterone

Gian Carlo Di Renzo [1,2,*], Valentina Tosto [1], Valentina Tsibizova [3] and Eduardo Fonseca [4]

1. Centre of Perinatal and Reproductive Medicine, Department of Obstetrics and Gynecology, University of Perugia, 06132 Perugia, Italy; tosto.valentina@libero.it
2. Department of Obstetrics and Gynecology, Faculty of General Medicine, I.M. Sechenov First State University of Moscow, 119991 Moscow, Russia
3. Almazov National Medical Research Centre, Health Ministry of Russian Federation, 197341 Saint Petersburg, Russia; tsibizova.v@gmail.com
4. Department of Obstetrics and Gynecology, Federal University of Paraiba, Joao Pessoa 58051-900, PB, Brazil; fonseca2003@yahoo.com
* Correspondence: giancarlo.direnzo@unipg.it

Abstract: Gestational age at birth is a critical factor for perinatal and adulthood outcomes, and even for transgenerational conditions' effects. Preterm birth (PTB) (prematurity) is still the main determinant for infant mortality and morbidity leading cause of infant morbidity and mortality. Unfortunately, preterm birth (PTB) is a relevant public health issue worldwide and the global PTB rate is around 11%. The premature activation of labor is underlined by complex mechanisms, with a multifactorial origin influenced by numerous known and probably unknown triggers. The possible mechanisms involved in a too early labor activation have been partially explained, and involve chemokines, receptors, and imbalanced inflammatory paths. Strategies for the early detection and prevention of this obstetric condition were proposed in clinical settings with interesting results. Progesterone has been demonstrated to have a key role in PTB prevention, showing several positive effects, such as lower prostaglandin synthesis, the inhibition of cervical stromal degradation, modulating the inflammatory response, reducing gap junction formation, and decreasing myometrial activation. The available scientific knowledge, data and recommendations address multiple current areas of debate regarding the use of progesterone in multifetal gestation, including different formulations, doses and routes of administration and its safety profile in pregnancy.

Keywords: preterm birth; risk factors; prevention; 17-OHPC; micronized progesterone; perinatal outcomes; recommendations

1. Introduction

Preterm birth is defined by the World Health Organization (WHO) as delivery before 37 completed weeks of gestation. About 85% of these premature births occur at 32 to 36 weeks, 10% are born at 28–31 weeks, and 5% at <28 weeks of gestation (extremely preterm babies).

Being born too soon is an important cause of infant deaths from prematurity every year, and many preterm newborns have long term disabilities. About 15 million babies are born preterm annually, with an increasing trend in cases rates worldwide, putting the global PTB rate at 11% [1–3].

There is growing evidence that the progesterone can be useful in high risk pregnancies for preterm birth. The use of progestogens has been extensively studied over the years and it is still a topic of interest in current research [4–13]. Expert researchers suggest that the rate of PTB may be reduced by the prophylactic use of progesterone, especially in women with a high risk profile, including a previous history of spontaneous preterm delivery and in women revealed to have a short cervical length (CL) at transvaginal ultrasound (TVU) [14].

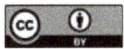

The complex pathogenesis of preterm labor activation makes reliable prediction difficult [15]. An obstetric history of spontaneous preterm birth (sPTB) is considered the strongest predicting factor. sPTB recurs in 35 to 50% of pregnancies, and the risk of a recurrent event recurrence is proportional to the number of prior spontaneous preterm deliveries. Several other risk factors have been associated with at the evidence surrounding the variability of this obstetric event, including non-Hispanic Black race, low socioeconomic status, midtrimester cervical length <25 mm, cervical-vaginal infections, history of cervical surgery procedures, maternal smoking, poor or no prenatal care, uterine overdistension, decidual hemorrhage, and short interpregnancy interval. Others conditions possibly associated with spontaneous preterm birth are multiple pregnancy, pregnancy derived by assisted reproductive techniques (ART), periodontal disease, maternal anemia, environmental factors and epigenetics [16]. Recently, experts advocated that a possible association may exist between environment and preterm birth. How pollution and other contaminants may induce maternal-fetal effects is still unexplained; however, some researchers have demonstrated the probable influence of air pollution on epigenetic effects. Other recent scientific evidence suggests that epigenetics may, in turn, be linked to preterm labor [17].

Table 1 lists the known risk factors, the level of association and the possible interventions for PTB.

Table 1. Risk factors, level of association with spontaneous PTB, available preventive-therapeutic interventions [15–22].

Risk Factors	Associations with Spontaneous PTB	Available Interventions
Ethnicity (black)	X	No
Maternal age (young age and advanced age)	X	Yes
Domestic violence	XX	Yes
Low socioeconomic status	XX	?
Stress, despression, negative life events	XX	Yes
Hard work	XX	Yes
No or poor prenatal care	XX	Yes
Smoking, substance abuse (cocaine)	X	Yes
Alcohol, caffeine	X	Yes
Pre-pregnancy BMI, weight gain in pregnancy	X	Yes
Previous preterm delivery or second trimester pregnancy loss	XXX	Yes
Previous cone biospy/cervix surgery	XX	?
Previous cesarean section	X	Yes
Mullerian abnormalities	X	No, Yes or ?
Parity (nulliparity?)	X	-
Short inter-pregnancy interval (<12 months)	X	Yes or ?
Family history for PTB, genetics	X	No
Male baby	X	No
Reproductive system disorders, treatments, ART	X	Yes
Maternal medical disorders (preeclampsia, diabetes, others)	X	No, Yes or ?
Multiple pregnancy	XXX	Yes
Vaginal bleeding	X	No or?
Cervico-vaginal infections	XX	Yes
Uterine contractility	X	Yes
Short cervix/Cervical modification (during antenatal surveillance)	XX	Yes
Periodontitis	X	Yes
Maternal anemia	X	Yes
Environmental factors and epigenetics	X	?

-: not applicable; PTB: preterm birth; ART: assisted reproductive technologies; BMI: body mass index; X: weak demonstrated association; XX: mild demonstrated association; XXX: strong demonstrated assoccation; ?: as-yet unidentified interventions.

Extensive data reported that the ultrasound measurement of CL at mid-gestation may be a useful strategy for predicting the risk of preterm birth delivery for both singleton and twin pregnancies [18–22]. A growing body of studies agree that the administration of progestogens to high-risk women, mainly with a singleton pregnancy, significantly reduces the rate of sPTB [4–8,23–25]. A lack of strong evidence and controversial opinions exist on progesterone's usefulness in twin/multifetal pregnancies.

2. Progesterone: Biochemical "Identikit" and Rationale for Use

The history of progesterone (PG) is long and characterized by numerous and fascinating chronological steps, and it is probably destinated to have a "never-ending history", as discussed in a recent paper [26,27]. Progesterone is probably the oldest hormone scientists know about. The terms "progestogens" or "progestagens" refer to natural or synthetic chemical forms with progestational activity.

Nowadays, the pharmacokinetic and pharmacodynamic features of progesterone are well-known.

The understanding of the pharmacodynamics of progesterone in preterm labor prevention is based on the evidence that it relaxes the uterus throughout pregnancy by inhibiting the expression of estrogen receptor alpha (ER-a) and reducing sensitivity to estrogen [28]. Overall, progesterone shows numerous functions on the myometrium: it has been shown to induce high levels of cyclic adenosine mono phosphate (cAMP) and time-dependent stimulation of nitric oxide synthetase (NOS), as well as to inhibit the myometrial gap junctions' (channels made of connexin 43) formation. Natural progesterone (P4) and its metabolites promote uterine quiescence both through interactions between nuclear and membrane P4 receptors and by inducing low levels of the inflammatory prostaglandins (via cyclooxygenase), oxytocin and intracellular calcium [29–32].

The route of administration seems crucial in determining the optimal pharmacodynamic profile of P4 and in obtaining the desired clinical effects. Most of the body of scientific evidence regards the vaginal, intramuscular and oral routes, as discussed below. The most important revolution in theme of progesterone is the development of micronization process, which led to further optimization of clinical effects and objectives deriving from its use. The micronization of progesterone and its suspension in oil-filled capsules was first studied in the late 1970s; this allowed progesterone to be absorbed more efficiently by the traditional oral route [26].

Nowadays, micronized progesterone products are largely preferred and used in obstetrics (and not only in this field) for many medical conditions, including threatened miscarriage, recurrent pregnancy loss and PTB prevention [26,33,34]. Based on the major part of consistent researches, the vaginal administration would be the best option to use due to the better concentrations that reach the uterus for the "first uterine pass effect" and to avoid the unwanted side effects such as nausea, headache, and sleepiness derived from oral route [26,35]. Table 2 reports the main e biochemical, immune and hormonal mechanisms of progesterone that are involved in the maintenance of pregnancy.

Table 2. Pharmacodynamic identikit of progesterone in pregnancy maintenance [26–32].

Biochemical, Immune and Hormonal Effects	+	−
Maternal immune responses modulation (fetus as semiallogenic transplant—needs protection)	+	
Utero-placental perfusion changes and improvements	+	
Myometrial/uterine relaxation through:	+	
-Estrogen receptors (ER-alpha) expression		−
-Estrogen sensitivity		−
-Oxytocin receptors antagonization		−
-Levels of cyclic adenosine mono phosphate (cAMP)	+	
-Nitric oxide synthetase (NOS)	+	
-Formation of myometrial gap junctions (channels made of connexin 43)		−
Cervix integrity promotion	+	
Suppression of fetal immunoplacental inflammatory response	+	
Cervix ripening		−
CRH (corticotrophin releasing hormone) and cortisol levels		−
Prostaglandins release		−
Vaginal microbiota influence (for vaginal administration)	+	

3. Progesterone and PTB: Where We Are Now

The current best approach to limit the preterm birth burden is based on early detection risk and prevention by multilevel and even combined strategies. In recent years, international and national societies have shown a great need to identify and manage women at risk of delivering prematurely, developing and sharing recommendations that are not absolute but which are, nevertheless, useful [36].

3.1. Identification of PTB High Risk Women

The traditional method of antenatal screening is based on an accurate history based on factors such as maternal age, race, smoking status, and previous and current obstetric history. The available risk scoring systems, which attempt to define the pregnancy's level of risk, have been shown to have a scarce detection rate and a high false-positive rate [37]. An alternative strategy is to identify high risk women by cervical length measurement at 20–24 weeks of gestation [14,18,19]. Studies revealed that in both singleton [14,18,19] and twin pregnancies [14] the rate of early spontaneous birth can be predicted from the measurement of CL in this gestational period.

Thus, measuring cervical length by TVU is a simple and effective test for the prevention of PTB, but routine CL screening is not clearly recommended by some international societies [37–41]. Furthermore, both the American College of Obstetricians and Gynecologists (ACOG) and the Society for Maternal–Fetal Medicine (SMFM) recognize that such a screening strategy may be considered [38–40].

The FIGO Working Group on Best Practice in maternal-fetal medicine was clear in its statement in favor of the universal screening of pregnant women by mid-trimester TVU evaluation of the cervical length as a useful intervention to decrease preterm births in pregnant women with a short cervix [36,42]. Similarly, the European Association of Perinatal Medicine had approved the universal CL screening as a relevant PTB detection strategy [43].

Once risk assessment is established, the choice on how to manage risk may involve one or a combination of several preventive strategies. Regarding progesterone use, differences exist worldwide.

3.2. Management of Short Cervix in Singleton Gestation with NO History of sPTB

Given the association of cervical shortening with preterm birth, several interventions aimed at decreasing the PTB rate have been investigated, including intramuscular 17-hydroxyprogesterone caproate (17-OHPC), cerclage, cervical pessary, and vaginal progesterone [9,44–47]. Studies of pessary and cerclage have produced conflicting results, while 17-OHCP treatment has failed to demonstrate benefit when prescribed for the indication of cervical shortening. The results have been consistently more beneficial and salutary for vaginal progesterone route. In a large multicenter trial, women with a cervical length <30 mm at 16 to 22 weeks were randomized to receive weekly injections of 17-OHPC or placebo. The rate of preterm delivery was similar between groups (25.1% vs. 24.2%, RR 1.03, 95% CI 0.79–1.35), and no improvement was seen in neonatal outcomes [45]. Two smaller studies produced conflicting results on the efficacy of 17-OHPC in the setting of short cervix, with one study demonstrating benefit similar to vaginal progesterone and the other demonstrating no advantage in preterm birth rate reduction. The efficacy of vaginal administration in women with a sonographic diagnosis of short cervix has been reported by two multicenter, randomized controlled trials and by independent patient-level meta-analyses that included data from these studies and several smaller trials. Fonseca et al. conducted a double-blind trial that randomized women with a cervical length ≤15 mm to 200 mg vaginal progesterone or placebo [5]. A total of 413 women were treated from 24 to 34 weeks' gestation. Delivery prior to 34 weeks was reduced to 19.2% in the group that received vaginal progesterone vs. 34.4% in the placebo group (RR 0.56, 95% CI 0.36–0.86). Eighty-five percent of the women included in this study had no history of preterm birth. In a subgroup analysis of these women, a relevant reduction in preterm birth rate at

<34 weeks was noted in women with a short cervix (≤15 mm) who received progesterone (RR 0.57, 95% CI 0.35–0.93) [5]. The PREGNANT trial reported that administration of vaginal progesterone gel (dose of 90 mg) in a pregnant group with a cervical length of 10 to 20 mm identified at mid-gestation resulted in a significant reduction in PTB rate at <33 weeks of gestation (8.9% vs. 16.1%, RR 0.55, 95% CI 0.33–0.92) [48]. Moreover, this study showed neonatal benefits, with a significant reduction in respiratory distress syndrome (RR 0.39, 95% CI 0.17–0.92). Only 16% of the enrolled population had a history of previous PTB, and even after excluding these subjects, progesterone remained associated with a relevant benefit in the setting of isolated short cervix (RR 0.50, 95% CI 0.27–0.90) [48]. A 2018 meta-analysis incorporated data on 974 singleton pregnancies with a CL ≤25 mm and described a decreased risk of preterm birth at <32 weeks of gestation (RR 0.64, 95% CI 0.48–0.86) with vaginal progesterone treatment; preterm deliveries at <28, <34, and <37 weeks of gestation were reduced as well. In addition, the meta-analysis showed a reduction in neonatal morbidity and mortality (RR 0.59, 95% CI 0.38–0.91), as well as a reduction in birthweight <2500 g and <1500 g [46]. Treatment with vaginal progesterone following the diagnosis of a short cervix and the threshold of cervical length at which to start treatment remain areas of debate. The US Food and Drug Administration (FDA) did not approve vaginal progesterone for the indication of preterm birth prevention in the setting of short CL, in part because data from the PREGNANT trial failed to demonstrate a benefit when only US patients were analyzed. In addition, the FDA declined approval because vaginal progesterone did not appear to be effective in Black or obese women. Despite debate about the clinical utility in all subgroups, given the data on the potential benefit and lack of harm, the ACOG and SMFM have recommended vaginal progesterone as a useful strategy for pregnant women with a short cervix [39]. In addition, with evidence of the benefits of vaginal progesterone administration in the setting of a short cervix and its cost-effectiveness, some experts have recommended universal cervical length screening for asymptomatic women without a prior preterm delivery [48–50]. The cost-effectiveness of such recommendations, however, is founded on a single, not serial, cervical length measurement at the time of mid-trimester ultrasound examination [51].

3.3. Management of Short Cervix in Singleton Gestation with History of sPTB

The National Institute of Child Health and Human Development (NICHD) Maternal–Fetal Medicine Units Network conducted a multicenter double-blind randomized controlled trial of 463 women with a singleton pregnancy and prior spontaneous preterm birth between 16 and 36 weeks who received 17-OHPC or placebo. Treatment with 17-OHPC was associated with a 34% reduction in recurrent preterm birth at <37 weeks of gestation (from 54.9 to 36.3%), as well as significant reductions at <32 and <35 weeks and decreased infant complications, such as intraventricular hemorrhage, necrotizing enterocolitis, and need for supplemental oxygen [13]. In 2011, the FDA approved 17-OHPC for prevention of recurrent preterm birth and it became the standard of care in the United States. More recently, research showed that 17-OHPC administration did not reduce the rate of preterm birth at <37 weeks of gestation (17-OHPC 11% vs. placebo 11.5%), nor did it reduce neonatal morbidity (5.6% vs. 5.0%) [52]. This study could not recruit well in the USA because 17-OHPC was already on the market and incorporated into the standard care for women with prior PTB, resulting in significant demographic and risk differences between the PROLONG trial and the NICHD study. Only 22% of patients enrolled in PROLONG were from the USA; 61% were from Russia and Ukraine. In addition, only 1.1% of patients had a cervical length <25 mm and only 7% of the patients were Black—two of the greatest risk factors for preterm birth. These differences in study populations and the conflicting results of the two trials have introduced considerable uncertainty and controversy into the management of patients with prior preterm birth with 17-OHPC. The FDA convened an advisory panel to review the data on 17-OHPC. The panel voted to recommend that the drug be removed from the market [53]. In October 2020, the FDA Center for Drug Evaluation and Research proposed withdrawal of 17-OHPC from the market. The final decision is subject to potential additional public hearings and a ruling from the FDA Commissioner [54].

A 2020 statement from SMFM concludes that providers can reasonably continue to use 17-OHPC in women with a risk profile similar to that of the enrollees in the NICHD study [55]. Given the preponderance of data in a USA population, the SMFM states that women with a singleton gestation and a history of prior sPTB may be prescribed intramuscular administration of 250 mg 17-OHPC weekly, starting at 16 to 20 weeks of gestation until 36 weeks of gestation or delivery. If 17-OHPC is not available or the patient declines this option, vaginal progesterone may be a reasonable alternative [55].

The clinical advantage of vaginal progesterone has been largely investigated and supported in women with prior spontaneous preterm delivery. While subsequent studies have produced mixed results, a 2019 meta-analysis readdressed the question of the optimal intervention for women with a prior preterm birth and confirmed that vaginal progesterone treatment was associated with a reduction in recurrent preterm birth at <34 weeks (OR 0.29, 95% CI 0.12–0.68) and <37 weeks (OR 0.43, 95% CI 0.23–0.74) [56].

At the present, the debate on intramuscular 17-OHPC, vaginal progesterone and which route and formulation is better is still open. The EPPPIC study group reported results of a meta-analysis, in which data from 31 trials were included. The authors considered trials of both singleton and multifetal pregnancies comparing vaginal, intramuscular and oral progesterone administration with control, or with each other. Compared with controls, both the vaginal route and the intramuscular 17-OHPC reduced the risk of PTB before 34 weeks for singleton pregnancies in high risk women, with a 22% reduction in the relative risk (RR) for participants who received vaginal progesterone (nine trials, 3769 women), and 17% reduction for those received 17-OHPC (five trials, 3053 women) [57]. Importantly, given that the upper confidence limit crosses the line of no effect, the reported implication that 17-hydroxyprogesterone caproate (17-OHPC) "reduced birth before 34 week in high-risk singleton pregnancies" is not justified in light of its lack of statistical significance. This erroneous conclusion could have serious consequences, as 17-OHCP does not have a good safety profile. It is well-established, including randomized evidence, that 17-OHCP causes gestational diabetes mellitus [58], a condition with adverse maternal and neonatal outcome. 17-OHCP is also associated with higher group B streptococcus (GBS) maternal colonization (a well-known contributor to neonatal morbidity and mortality) compared to vaginal progesterone administration [59]. There is also a known increase of cancer in the offspring of mothers treated with 17-OHCP, as reported at the Endocrine Society's recent annual conference [60].

Regarding the utility of oral progesterone administration as preventive strategy in high risk patients, evidence to support its use in clinical routine practice is still inconsistent [57].

A recent study reported that oral progesterone appears to be effective for the prevention of recurrent preterm delivery and reduction in perinatal morbidity and mortality in asymptomatic singleton pregnancies compared with placebo. More adverse effects with oral progesterone therapy compared with placebo were reported, although none were serious. Thus, future randomized studies comparing oral progesterone with other available therapies for the prevention of recurrent preterm birth are needed [61].

3.4. Multiple Pregnancy

Twin pregnancies are associated with a several-fold greater perinatal mortality than singleton pregnancies. PTB Prematurity is an important contributor, with about 50% of twin pregnancies delivering before 37 weeks and 10% delivering before 32 weeks [62]. Trials in unselected twin pregnancies reported that use of progesterone from mid gestation had no relevant effect on reducing prematurity for twins. Just recently, a multicenter trial conducted at 22 European hospitals was published. Women with twin pregnancy were randomly assigned to receive either progesterone (early administration of 600 mcg/daily vaginal progesterone from 11 to 14 weeks) or placebo, and in the random-sequence generation, there was stratification according to the participating center. The results reveal that universal treatment with vaginal progesterone does not reduce the incidence of spontaneous birth between 24^{+0} and 33^{+6} weeks' gestation. Post hoc time-to-event analysis led to the suggestion that progesterone may reduce the risk of spontaneous birth before 32 weeks' gestation in women with a cervical length of <30 mm, and it may increase the risk for those with a cervical length of ≥30 mm [63]. In conclusion, there is no strong evidence of the benefit of using universal vaginal progesterone to decrease prematurity in multiple pregnancies. One meta-analysis showed a benefit in reducing adverse perinatal outcomes in a subgroup of women with a short cervix ≤25 mm, suggesting it may be useful in this group, but the study design had several limits and further research is needed. The NICE guidelines for multiple pregnancy followed by UK healthcare providers do not promote the routine use of cervical cerclage or progesterone for the prevention of PTB in multiple pregnancies.

3.5. Combination of Preventive and Therapeutic Strategies

Data regarding the efficacy of combining different approaches, such as intramuscular progesterone with or without vaginal progesterone and with or without cervical cerclage and Arabin pessary, are limited, not unanimous, but in evolution. The utility of combined treatment with history-based cerclage and intramuscular 17-OHPC is unclear, and small retrospective studies have reported mixed results [64,65]. The SMFM recommends continuation of 17-OHPC in women who receive an ultrasound-indicated cerclage [66]. Most recently, Shor et al. said that a combined rescue therapy including vaginal progesterone, cervical cerclage, and Arabin cervical pessary emerges as a promising management strategy in pregnant women who have a short cervical length and a high background risk for preterm delivery [67]. The possible advantages of a combined approach were also considered for twin pregnancies. In this regard, a recent study evaluated the efficacy of a combined approach (vaginal progesterone plus cervical pessary) and of vaginal progesterone only in twin pregnancies: the combined use of Arabin cervical pessary and vaginal progesterone in twin pregnancy with short CL may have a synergic and beneficial effect in preventing preterm labor [68]. On the opposite, D'Antonio et al. observed that cervical pessary, progesterone and cerclage do not show a significant effect in reducing the rate of PTB or perinatal morbidity in twins, either when these strategies are applied to an unselected population of twins or in pregnancies with a short cervix [69]. Further research is needed to confirm whether or not these preliminary data both in singleton and twin pregnancies.

4. Progesterone Safety Profile

The safety profile of progesterone on newborn health is another topic of growing interest among experts. Many questions remain unexplained, particularly the long-term safety concerns and also whether the use of progestagens may or not improve neonatal and childhood outcomes.

The results of a meta-analysis suggest that the administration of progestogen for preterm birth prevention does not appear to negatively affect neonatal mortality in single or multiple pregnancies regardless of the route of administration [70]. Moreover, similar conclusions were derived from a study on twins, in which the authors found that antenatal exposure to progesterone given in twin pregnancies has no significant impact on child health and developmental outcomes at three to six years [71].

A recent systematic review examined the potential long-term effects of prenatal progesterone treatment on child development, behavior and health: the authors did not find evidence of benefit or harm in offspring prenatally exposed to progesterone treatment for PTB prevention [72]. There is a need for future follow-up studies on prenatal progesterone administration and its effects in offspring beyond early childhood. Therefore, nowadays, the safety profile of natural progesterone is quite confirmed, while the one of progestogens is raising many issues of concern (particularly relating to the use of 17-OHPC and dydrogesterone as alternatives to natural progesterone) [32,35,60].

5. Conclusions

The current scientific and clinical evidence suggest that cervical length screening and vaginal progesterone use, eventually combined with cervical cerclage or Arabin pessary, may help to contain or reduce the burden of preterm delivery birth, when used in the appropriate target populations of pregnant women. The current data and recommendations address multiple controversial topic areas regarding the role of progesterone for PTB prevention in multi-gestational pregnancies multifetal gestation, its different formulations, dosages, routes of administration and safety profile in pregnancy. Overall, a growing body of studies are in agreement in identifying progesterone, especially the vaginal formulation, as a keystone among the preventive PTB strategies in well-defined high-risk categories.

Author Contributions: Conceptualization, G.C.D.R.; methodology, V.T. (Valentina Tosto) and V.T. (Valentina Tsibizova); validation, G.C.D.R. and E.F.; formal analysis, G.C.D.R.; investigation, V.T. (Valentina Tosto), V.T. (Valentina Tsibizova) and E.F.; resources, G.C.D.R.; data curation, G.C.D.R.; writing—original draft preparation, G.C.D.R. and E.F.; writing—review and editing, G.C.D.R., V.T. (Valentina Tosto) and E.F.; visualization, G.C.D.R.; supervision, G.C.D.R.; No need of project administration; No funding acquisition. All authors have read and agreed to the published version of the manuscript.

Funding: This research received no external funding.

Data Availability Statement: The data presented in this paper are available in public datasets at doi, reference number.

Conflicts of Interest: The authors declare no conflict of interest.

References

1. Blencowe, H.; Cousens, S.; Oestergaard, M.Z.; Chou, D.; Moller, A.-B.; Narwal, R.; Adler, A.; Garcia, C.V.; Rohde, S.; Say, L.; et al. National, regional, and worldwide estimates of preterm birth rates in the year 2010 with time trends since 1990 for selected countries: A systematic analysis and implications. *Lancet* **2012**, *379*, 2162–2172. [CrossRef]
2. Chang, H.H.; Larson, J.; Blencowe, H.; Spong, C.Y.; Howson, C.P.; Cairns-Smith, S.; Lackritz, E.M.; Lee, S.K.; Mason, E.; Serazin, A.C.; et al. Preventing preterm births: Analysis of trends and potential reductions with interventions in 39 countries with very high human development index. *Lancet* **2012**, *381*, 223–234. [CrossRef]
3. Torchin, H.; Ancel, P.Y.; Jarreau, P.H.; Goffinet, F. Epidemiology of preterm birth: Prevalence, recent trends, short- and longterm outcomes. *J. Gynecol. Obstet. Biol. Reprod.* **2015**, *44*, 723–731. [CrossRef] [PubMed]
4. Sanchez-Ramos, L.; Kaunitz, A.M.; Delke, I. Progestational agents to prevent preterm birth: A meta-analysis of randomized con-trolled trials. *Obstet. Gynecol.* **2005**, *105*, 273–279. [CrossRef] [PubMed]
5. Fonseca, E.B.; Celik, E.; Parra, M.; Singh, M.; Nicolaides, K.H. Progesterone and the Risk of Preterm Birth among Women with a Short Cervix. *N. Engl. J. Med.* **2007**, *357*, 462–469. [CrossRef] [PubMed]
6. DeFranco, E.A.; O'Brien, J.M.; Adair, C.D.; Lewis, D.F.; Hall, D.R.; Fusey, S.; Soma-Pillay, P.; Porter, K.; How, H.; Schakis, R.; et al. Vaginal progesterone is associated with a decrease in risk for early preterm birth and improved neonatal outcome in women with a short cervix: A secondary analysis from a randomized, double-blind, placebo-controlled trial. *Ultrasound Obstet. Gynecol.* **2007**, *30*, 697–705. [CrossRef]
7. Dodd, J.M.; Flenady, V.; Cincotta, R.; Crowther, C.A.; Windrim, R.C.; Kingdom, J.P. Progesterone for the prevention of preterm birth: A systematic review. *Obstet. Gynecol.* **2008**, *112*, 127–134. [CrossRef]
8. Keirse, M.J.N.C. Progestogen administration in pregnancy may prevent preterm delivery. *BJOG Int. J. Obstet. Gynaecol.* **1990**, *97*, 149–154. [CrossRef]
9. Hassan, S.S.; Romero, R.; Vidyadhari, D.; Fusey, S.; Baxter, J.K.; Khandelwal, M.; Vijayaraghavan, J.; Trivedi, Y.; Soma-Pillay, P.; Sambarey, P.; et al. Vaginal progesterone reduces the rate of preterm birth in women with a sonographic short cervix: A multicenter, randomized, double-blind, placebo-controlled trial. *Ultrasound Obstet. Gynecol.* **2011**, *38*, 18–31. [CrossRef]
10. Dodd, J.M.; Jones, L.; Flenady, V.; Cincotta, R.; Crowther, C.A. Prenatal administration of progesterone for preventing preterm birth in women considered to be at risk of preterm birth. *Cochrane Database Syst. Rev.* **2013**, CD004947. [CrossRef]
11. Cetingoz, E.; Cam, C.; Sakalli, M.; Karateke, A.; Çelik, C.; Sancak, A.; Sakallı, M. Progesterone effects on preterm birth in high-risk pregnancies: A randomized placebo-controlled trial. *Arch. Gynecol. Obstet.* **2010**, *283*, 423–429. [CrossRef]
12. da Fonseca, E.B.; Bittar, R.E.; Carvalho, M.H.; Zugaib, M. Prophylactic administration of progesterone by vaginal suppository to reduce the incidence of spontaneous preterm birth in women at increased risk: A randomized placebo-controlled doubleblind study. *Am. J. Obstet. Gynecol.* **2003**, *188*, 419–424. [CrossRef]

13. Meis, P.J.; Klebanoff, M.; Thom, E.; Dombrowski, M.P.; Sibai, B.; Moawad, A.H.; Spong, C.Y.; Hauth, J.C.; Miodovnik, M.; Varn23er, M.; et al. Prevention of Recurrent Preterm Delivery by 17 Alpha-Hydroxyprogesterone Caproate. *N. Engl. J. Med.* **2003**, *348*, 2379–2385. [CrossRef]
14. da Fonseca, E.B.; Damião, R.; Moreira, D.A. Preterm birth prevention. *Best Pract. Res. Clin. Obstet. Gynaecol.* **2020**, *69*, 40–49.
15. Di Renzo, G.C.; Tosto, V.; Giardina, I. The biological basis and prevention of preterm birth. *Best Pactr. Res. Clin. Obstet. Gynaecol.* **2018**, *52*, 13–22. [CrossRef]
16. Ferraro, D.M.; Larson, J.; Jacobsonn, B.; Di Renzo, G.C.; Norman, J.E.; Martin, J.N., Jr.; D'Alton, M.; Castelazo, E.; Howson, C.P.; Sengpiel, V.; et al. Cross-Country Individual Participant Analysis of 4.1 Million Singleton Births in 5 Countries with Very High Human Development Index Confirms Known Associations but Provides No Biologic Explanation for 2/3 of All Preterm Births. *PLoS ONE* **2016**, *11*, e0162506. [CrossRef] [PubMed]
17. Lin, V.W.; Baccarelli, A.A.; Burris, H.H. Epigenetics—A potential mediator between air pollution and preterm birth. *Environ. Epigenetics* **2016**, *2*. [CrossRef] [PubMed]
18. Celik, E.; To, M.; Gajewska, K.; Smith, G.C.S.; Nicolaides, K.H.; On behalf of the Fetal Medicine Foundation Second Trimester Screening Group. Cervical length and obstetric history predict spontaneous preterm birth: Development and validation of a model to provide individualized risk assessment. *Ultrasound Obstet. Gynecol.* **2008**, *31*, 549–554.
19. Berghella, V. Novel developments on cervical length screening and progesterone for preventing preterm birth. *BJOG Int. J. Obstet. Gynaecol.* **2008**, *116*, 182–187. [CrossRef]
20. To, M.S.; Skentou, C.A.; Royston, P.; Yu, C.K.H.; Nicolaides, K. Prediction of patient-specific risk of early preterm delivery using maternal history and sonographic measurement of cervical length: A population-based prospective study. *Ultrasound Obstet. Gynecol.* **2006**, *27*, 362–367. [CrossRef] [PubMed]
21. Berghella, V.; Roman, A.; Daskalakis, C.; Ness, A.; Baxter, J.K. Gestational age at cervical length measurement and incidence of preterm birth. *Obstet. Gynecol.* **2007**, *110*, 311–317. [CrossRef] [PubMed]
22. To, M.S.; Fonseca, E.B.; Molina, F.S.; Cacho, A.M.; Nicolaides, K.H. Maternal characteristics and cervical length in the prediction of spontaneous early preterm delivery in twins. *Am. J. Obstet. Gynecol.* **2006**, *194*, 1360–1365. [CrossRef] [PubMed]
23. Di Renzo, G.C.; Giardina, I.; Clerici, G.; Brillo, E.; Gerli, S. Progesterone in normal and pathological pregnancy. *Horm. Mol. Biol. Clin. Investig.* **2016**, *27*, 35–48. [CrossRef] [PubMed]
24. da Fonseca, E.B.; Damião, R.; Nicholaides, K. Prevention of Preterm Birth Based on Short Cervix: Progesterone. *Semin. Perinatol.* **2009**, *33*, 334–337. [CrossRef] [PubMed]
25. da Fonseca, E.B.; Bittar, R.E.; Damião, R.; Zugaib, M. Prematurity prevention: The role of progesterone. *Curr. Opin. Obstet. Gynecol.* **2009**, *21*, 142–147. [CrossRef] [PubMed]
26. Di Renzo, G.C.; Tosto, V.; Tsibizova, V. Progesterone: History, facts and artifacts. *Best Pract. Res. Clin. Obstet. Gynaecol.* **2020**, *69*, 2–12. [CrossRef] [PubMed]
27. Piette, P. The history of natural progesterone, the never-ending story. *Climacteric* **2018**, *21*, 308–314. [CrossRef]
28. Mesiano, S.; Chan, E.-C.; Fitter, J.T.; Kwek, K.; Yeo, G.; Smith, R. Progesterone Withdrawal and Estrogen Activation in Human Parturition are Coordinated by Progesterone Receptor A Expression in the Myometrium. *J. Clin. Endocrinol. Metab.* **2002**, *87*, 2924–2930. [CrossRef]
29. Pierce, B.T.; Calhoun, B.C.; Adolphson, K.R.; Lau, A.F.; Pierce, L.M. Connexin 43 expression in normal versus prolonged labor. *Am. J. Obstet. Gynecol.* **2002**, *186*, 504–511. [CrossRef]
30. Cluff, A.H.; Bystrom, B.; Klimaviciute, A.; Dahlqvist, C.; Cebers, G.; Malmstrom, A.; Ekman-Ordeberg, G. Prolonged labour associated with lower expression of syndecan 3 and connexin 43 in human uterine tissue. *Reprod. Biol. Endocrinol.* **2006**, *4*, 24. [CrossRef]
31. Spong, C.Y. Prediction and prevention of recurrent spontaneous preterm birth. *Obstet. Gynecol.* **2007**, *110*, 405–415. [CrossRef]
32. Piette, P.C. The pharmacodynamics and safety of progesterone. *Best Pract. Res. Clin. Obstet. Gynaecol.* **2020**, *69*, 13–29. [CrossRef]
33. Di Renzo, G.C.; Fonseca, E. Re: Effect of progestogen for women with threatened miscarriage: A systematic review and meta-analysis. *BJOG Int. J. Obstet. Gynaecol.* **2020**, *127*, 1304–1305. [CrossRef] [PubMed]
34. Coomarasamy, A.; Devall, A.J.; Brosens, J.J.; Quenby, S.; Stephenson, M.D.; Sierra, S.; Christiansen, O.B.; Small, R.; Brewin, J.; Roberts, T.E.; et al. Micronized vaginal progesterone to prevent miscarriage: A critical evaluation of randomized evidence. *Am. J. Obstet. Gynecol.* **2020**, *223*, 167–176. [CrossRef] [PubMed]
35. Di Renzo, G.C. Concerns about the review of vaginal progesterone and the vaginal first-pass effect. *Climacteric* **2019**, *22*, 105. [CrossRef] [PubMed]
36. FIGO Working Group on Good Clinical Practice in Maternal–Fetal Medicine; Di Renzo, G.C.; Fonseca, E.; Gratacos, E.; Hassan, S.; Kurtser, M.; Malone, F.; Nambiar, S.; Nicolaides, K.; Sierra, N.; et al. Good clinical practice advice: Prediction of preterm labor and preterm premature rupture of membranes. *Int. J. Gynecol. Obstet.* **2018**, *144*, 340–346.
37. Honest, H.; Bachmann, L.; Sundaram, R.; Gupta, J.; Kleijnen, J.; Khan, K. The accuracy of risk scores in predicting preterm birth—A systematic review. *J. Obstet. Gynaecol.* **2004**, *24*, 343–359. [CrossRef] [PubMed]
38. American College of Obstetricians and Gynecologists. ACOG Committee Opinion: Use of progesterone to reduce preterm birth. *Obstet. Gynecol.* **2008**, *419*, 963–965. [CrossRef]
39. Committee on Practice Bulletins—Obstetrics, The American College of Obstetricians and Gynecologists. Practice bulletin no. 130: Prediction and prevention of preterm birth. *Obstet. Gynecol.* **2012**, *120*, 964–973. [CrossRef]

40. Society for Maternal-Fetal Medicine Publications Committee, with assistance of Vincenzo Berghella. Progesterone and preterm birth prevention: Translating clinical trials data into clinical practice. *Am. J. Obstet. Gynecol.* **2012**, *206*, 376–386. [CrossRef]
41. Lim, K.; Butt, K.; Crane, J.M. No. 257-Ultrasonographic cervical length assessment in predicting preterm birth in singleton pregnancies. *J. Obstet. Gynaecol. Can.* **2018**, *40*, e151–e164. [CrossRef]
42. Figo Working Group on Best Practice in Maternal-Fetal Medicine, International Federation of Gynecology and Obstetrics. Best practice in maternal-fetal medicine. *Int. J. Gynecol. Obstet.* **2015**, *128*, 80–82. [CrossRef]
43. Di Renzo, G.C.; Roura, L.C.; Facchinetti, F.; Helmer, H.; Hubinont, C.; Jacobsson, B.; Jørgensen, J.S.; Lamont, R.F.; Mikhailov, A.; Papantoniou, N.; et al. Preterm Labor and Birth Management: Recommendations from the European Association of Perinatal Medicine. *J. Matern. Neonatal Med.* **2017**, *30*, 2011–2030. [CrossRef] [PubMed]
44. Goya, M.; Pratcorona, L.; Merced, C.; Rodó, C.; Valle, L.; Romero, A.; Juan, M.; Rodríguez, A.; Muñoz, B.; Santacruz, B.; et al. Cervical pessary in pregnant women with a short cervix (PECEP): An open-label randomised controlled trial. *Lancet* **2012**, *379*, 1800–1806. [CrossRef]
45. Grobman, W.A.; Thom, E.A.; Spong, C.Y.; Iams, J.D.; Saade, G.R.; Mercer, B.M.; Tita, A.; Rouse, D.J.; Sorokin, Y.; Wapner, R.; et al. 17 alpha-hydroxyprogesterone caproate to prevent prematurity in nulliparas with cervical length less than 30 mm. *Am. J. Obstet. Gynecol.* **2012**, *207*, 390.e1–390.e8. [CrossRef] [PubMed]
46. Romero, R.; Conde-Agudelo, A.; Da Fonseca, E.; O'Brien, J.M.; Cetingoz, E.; Creasy, G.W.; Hassan, S.S.; Nicolaides, K. Vaginal progesterone for preventing preterm birth and adverse perinatal outcomes in singleton gestations with a short cervix: A meta-analysis of individual patient data. *Am. J. Obstet. Gynecol.* **2018**, *218*, 161–180. [CrossRef] [PubMed]
47. Romero, R.; Conde-Agudelo, A.; El-Refaie, W.; Rode, L.; Brizot, M.L.; Cetingoz, E.; Serra, V.; Da Fonseca, E.; Abdelhafez, M.; Tabor, A.; et al. Vaginal progesterone decreases preterm birth and neonatal morbidity and mortality in women with a twin gestation and a short cervix: An updated meta-analysis of individual patient data. *Ultrasound Obstet. Gynecol.* **2017**, *49*, 303–314. [CrossRef] [PubMed]
48. Einerson, B.D.; Grobman, W.A.; Miller, E.S. Cost-effectiveness of risk-based screening for cervical length to prevent preterm birth. *Am. J. Obstet. Gynecol.* **2016**, *215*, 100.e1–100.e7. [CrossRef] [PubMed]
49. Cahill, A.G.; Odibo, A.O.; Caughey, A.B.; Stamilio, D.M.; Hassan, S.S.; Macones, G.A.; Romero, R. Universal cervical length screening and treatment with vaginal progesterone to prevent preterm birth: A decision and economic analysis. *Am. J. Obstet. Gynecol.* **2010**, *202*, 548.e1–548.e8. [CrossRef] [PubMed]
50. Werner, E.F.; Hamel, M.S.; Orzechowski, K.; Berghella, V.; Thung, S.F. Cost-effectiveness of transvaginal ultrasound cervical length screening in singletons without a prior preterm birth: An update. *Am. J. Obstet. Gynecol.* **2015**, *213*, 554.e1–554.e6. [CrossRef]
51. Biggio, J.R. Current Approaches to Risk Assessment and Prevention of Preterm Birth—A Continuing Public Health Crisis. *Ochsner J.* **2020**, *20*, 426–433. [CrossRef]
52. Blackwell, S.C.; Gyamfi-Bannerman, C.; Biggio, J.R.; Chauhan, S.P.; Hughes, B.L.; Louis, J.; Manuck, T.A.; Miller, H.S.; Das, A.F.; Saade, G.R.; et al. 17-OHPC to Prevent Recurrent Preterm Birth in Singleton Gestations (PROLONG Study): A Multicenter, International, Randomized Double-Blind Trial. *Am. J. Perinatol.* **2019**, *37*, 127–136. [CrossRef]
53. FDA Advisory board Votes to Recommend Withdrawing Progesterone Therapy for Preterm birth. Pharmacy Times. 30 October 2019. Available online: www.pharmacytimes.com/news/fda-advisory-board-votes-to-recommend-withdrawing-progesterone-therapy-for-preterm-birth (accessed on 22 October 2020).
54. CDER Proposes Withdrawal of Approval for Makena. U.S. Food and Drug Administration. Available online: www.fda.gov/drugs/drug-safety-and-availability/cder-proposes-withdrawal-approval-makena (accessed on 22 October 2020).
55. Society for Maternal-Fetal Medicine (SMFM) Publications Committee. SMFM Statement: Use of 17-alpha hydroxyprogesterone caproate for prevention of recurrent preterm birth. *Am. J. Obstet. Gynecol.* **2020**, *223*, B16–B18. [CrossRef]
56. Jarde, A.; Lutsiv, O.; Beyene, J.; McDonald, S.D. Vaginal progesterone, oral progesterone, 17-OHPC, cerclage, and pessary for preventing preterm birth in at-risk singleton pregnancies: An updated systematic review and network meta-analysis. *BJOG Int. J. Obstet. Gynaecol.* **2018**, *126*, 556–567. [CrossRef]
57. Stewart, L.A.; Simmonds, M.; Duley, L.; Llewellyn, A.; Sharif, S.; Walker, R.A.; Beresford, L.; Wright, K.; Aboulghar, M.M.; Alfirevic, Z.; et al. Evaluating Progestogens for Preventing Preterm birth International Collaborative (EPPPIC): Meta-analysis of individual participant data from randomised controlled trials. *Lancet* **2021**, *397*, 1183–1194. [CrossRef]
58. Egerman, R.; Ramsey, R.; Istwan, N.; Rhea, D.; Stanziano, G. Maternal Characteristics Influencing the Development of Gestational Diabetes in Obese Women Receiving 17-alpha-Hydroxyprogesterone Caproate. *J. Obes.* **2014**, *2014*, 563243. [CrossRef] [PubMed]
59. Ma'Ayeh, M.; Rood, K.; Walker, H.; Oliver, E.; Gee, S.; Iams, J. Vaginal progesterone is associated with decreased group B streptococcus colonisation at term: A retrospective cohort study. *BJOG Int. J. Obstet. Gynaecol.* **2019**, *126*, 1141–1147. [CrossRef] [PubMed]
60. Hydroxyprogesterone Caproate May Contribute to Increasing Rates of Early-Onset Cancer, Researchers Say. Available online: https://www.endocrine.org (accessed on 11 March 2021).
61. Boelig, R.C.; Della Corte, L.; Ashoush, S.; McKenna, D.; Saccone, G.; Rajaram, S.; Berghella, V. Oral progesterone for the prevention of recurrent preterm birth: Systematic review and metaanalysis. *Am. J. Obstet. Gynecol. MFM* **2019**, *1*, 50–62. [CrossRef] [PubMed]
62. Murray, S.R.; Stock, S.J.; Cowan, S.; Cooper, E.S.; Norman, J. Spontaneous preterm birth prevention in multiple pregnancy. *Obstet. Gynaecol.* **2018**, *20*, 57–63. [CrossRef]

63. Rehal, A.; Benkő, Z.; Matallana, C.D.P.; Syngelaki, A.; Janga, D.; Cicero, S.; Akolekar, R.; Singh, M.; Chaveeva, P.; Burgos, J.; et al. Early vaginal progesterone versus placebo in twin pregnancies for the prevention of spontaneous preterm birth: A randomized, double-blind trial. *Am. J. Obstet. Gynecol.* **2020**, *224*, 86.e1–86.e19. [CrossRef]
64. Rafael, T.J.; Zavodnick, J.; Berghella, V.; Mackeen, A.D. Effectiveness of 17-α-Hydroxyprogesterone Caproate on Preterm Birth Prevention in Women with History-Indicated Cerclage. *Am. J. Perinatol.* **2013**, *30*, 755–758. [CrossRef]
65. Stetson, B.; Hibbard, J.U.; Wilkins, I.; Leftwich, H. Outcomes with Cerclage Alone Compared with Cerclage Plus 17α-Hydroxyprogesterone Caproate. *Obstet. Gynecol.* **2016**, *128*, 983–988. [CrossRef] [PubMed]
66. SMFM preterm birth toolkit. Society for Maternal-Fetal Medicine. 2016. Available online: www.smfm.org/publications/231-smfm-preterm-birth-toolkit (accessed on 22 October 2020).
67. Shor, S.; Zimerman, A.; Maymon, R.; Kovo, M.; Wolf, M.; Wiener, I.; Bar, J.; Melcer, Y. Combined therapy with vaginal progesterone, Arabin cervical pessary and cervical cerclage to prevent preterm delivery in high-risk women. *J. Matern. Neonatal Med.* **2019**, *34*, 2154–2158. [CrossRef] [PubMed]
68. Yaniv-Nachmani, H.; Melcer, Y.; Weiner, I.; Bar, K.; Kovo, M.; Hershko, C.; Wolf, M.F.; Zimerman, A.; Maymon, R. A comparison of arabin cervical pessary and vaginal progesterone versus vaginal progesterone only in twin pregnancy for the prevention of preterm birth due to short cervix. *Harefuah* **2021**, *160*, 13–18. [PubMed]
69. D'Antonio, F.; Berghella, V.; Di Mascio, D.; Saccone, G.; Sileo, F.; Flacco, M.E.; Odibo, A.O.; Liberati, M.; Manzoli, L.; Khalil, A. Role of progesterone, cerclage and pessary in preventing preterm birth in twin pregnancies: A systematic review and network meta-analysis. *Eur. J. Obstet. Gynecol. Reprod. Biol.* **2021**, *261*, 166–177. [CrossRef] [PubMed]
70. Ahn, K.O.; Bae, N.-Y.; Hong, S.-C.; Lee, J.-S.; Lee, E.H.; Jee, H.-J.; Cho, G.-J.; Oh, M.-J.; Kim, H.-J. The safety of progestogen in the prevention of preterm birth: Meta-analysis of neonatal mortality. *J. Perinat. Med.* **2017**, *45*, 11–20. [CrossRef] [PubMed]
71. McNamara, H.C.; Wood, R.; Chalmers, J.; Marlow, N.; Norrie, J.; MacLennan, G.; McPherson, G.; Boachie, C.; Norman, J.E. STOPPIT Baby Follow-Up Study: The Effect of Prophylactic Progesterone in Twin Pregnancy on Childhood Outcome. *PLoS ONE* **2015**, *10*, e0122341.
72. Simons, N.E.; Leeuw, M.; Hooft, J.V.; Limpens, J.; Roseboom, T.J.; Oudijk, M.A.; Pajkrt, E.; Finken, M.J.; Painter, R.C. The long-term effect of prenatal progesterone treatment on child development, behaviour and health: A systematic review. *BJOG Int. J. Obstet. Gynaecol.* **2020**, *128*, 964–974. [CrossRef]

MDPI
St. Alban-Anlage 66
4052 Basel
Switzerland
Tel. +41 61 683 77 34
Fax +41 61 302 89 18
www.mdpi.com

Journal of Clinical Medicine Editorial Office
E-mail: jcm@mdpi.com
www.mdpi.com/journal/jcm

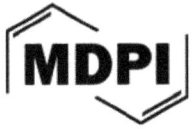